Brief Therapy for Clients with Challenging or Unique Issues

Brief Therapy for Clients with Challenging or Unique Issues offers clinicians, interns, and students a unique look into the creative and effective application of foundational concepts and innovative clinical processes that lead to successful outcomes for even the most challenging clients. Chapters illustrate complex interventions such as those involving clients court ordered or coerced into therapy; first-generation immigrant families in the criminal justice system; families at risk of losing custody of their children; foster children in the child welfare system; clients of multigenerational poverty; families requiring in-home family therapy; and more. Each of these includes moment-by-moment co-constructive processes that document effective intervention ideas and strategies.

Rich in neurolinguistics, innovative approaches, and the application of advanced solution-oriented strategies, *Brief Therapy for Clients with Challenging or Unique Issues* weaves together the stories of courageous clients and offers innovative tools that empower and motivate even the most reluctant clients to engage and identify solutions that fit for them.

Saul A. Singer, LMFT, LCADC, AADC, has worked for five decades as a behavioral health and addiction professional providing therapy, consultation, continuing education, college instruction, and clinical supervision in private practice and for community agencies and treatment programs.

Brief Therapy for Clients with Challenging or Unique Issues

A Clinician's Guide to Enhancing Outcomes

Saul A. Singer

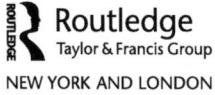
Routledge
Taylor & Francis Group

NEW YORK AND LONDON

Designed cover image: master1305 © Getty Images

First published 2024
by Routledge
605 Third Avenue, New York, NY 10158

and by Routledge
4 Park Square, Milton Park, Abingdon, Oxon, OX14 4RN

Routledge is an imprint of the Taylor & Francis Group, an informa business

Library of Congress Cataloging-in-Publication Data
Names: Singer, Saul A. (Psychotherapist), author.
Title: Brief therapy for clients with challenging or unique issues :
a clinician's guide to enhancing outcomes / Saul A. Singer.
Description: New York, NY : Routledge, 2024. |
Includes bibliographical references and index. |
Identifiers: LCCN 2023015127 (print) | LCCN 2023015128 (ebook) |
ISBN 9781032492438 (hardback) | ISBN 9781032492421 (paperback) |
ISBN 9781003397380 (ebook)
Subjects: LCSH: Brief psychotherapy. | Brief psychotherapy–Case studies.
Classification: LCC RC480.55 .S5727 2024 (print) |
LCC RC480.55 (ebook) | DDC 616.89/147–dc23/eng/20230623
LC record available at https://lccn.loc.gov/2023015127
LC ebook record available at https://lccn.loc.gov/2023015128

ISBN: 9781032492438 (hbk)
ISBN: 9781032492421 (pbk)
ISBN: 9781003397380 (ebk)

DOI: 10.4324/9781003397380

Typeset in Sabon
by Newgen Publishing UK

I am thankful to many for their assistance and support over the years: mentors, clients, friends, and family, including my children Monica, Mark, Jonathan, and Caroline; and most notably my wife, Barbara, whose saintly patience, encouragement, and top-notch proofreading made this work possible.

Contents

Prologue: Eyes Wide Open

Over the years, again and again, I have witnessed clients expressing strategic ideas and solutions to challenges even before they themselves realize that they have the answers. As clinicians, too often we minimize clients' strengths, courage, determination, and resilience, and put ourselves in the expert's seat. Much of our training involves clinical models that give us a false sense of control over process and change, and reliance on a structured intervention can cause us to lose sight of each client's unique assets. The ability to tap into a client's strengths, creativity, and unique change process is a core clinical skill necessary to facilitate the permanent change sought by the client.

Through the eyes of a seasoned psychotherapist in clinical practice for five decades, this book presents an accurate, sometimes verbatim account of how collaborating with and eliciting the knowledge of the client is the primary tool in facilitating desired change. Successful clinical practice in the real world is more about unmasking and applying client knowledge and wisdom than about telling the client what to do. Permanent change rarely, if ever, comes about from being told what to do or what not to do. When we become skilled at engagement—hearing a client's clear priorities, eliciting the client's solutions, and co-constructing what the client wants—we can sow the seeds for an internal change process to blossom.

In the clinical world, there are many ideas, models, and approaches that work at least somewhat with some clients; but they are often based on deficits and may rely on the clinician to be the expert in the therapeutic relationship. We need to know better. We need to do better. Any structured clinical approach will have limitations that hinder both engagement and successful outcomes for large swaths of the client population. Opportunities are lost when clinicians become rigid and driven by a clinical model or approach that is not a good fit for a particular client, and then blames the client if engagement or therapy is not effective. Especially for reluctant clients, therapy can feel like drudgery and seem designed to be intimidating or even hurtful.

Allowing the client to be the expert on their domain, and putting the responsibility for and mechanisms of change in their hands, will more often result in meaningful and lasting change, eliminate resistance, and reduce recidivism. One benefit to the clinician will be that therapy is more enjoyable and successful. Let's face it: clients are the real experts on their own lives and are in charge of change. Whenever the clinician assumes the role as the "advisor" or "expert" in the therapeutic relationship, there will be limitations in engagement and outcome; and too often, change will not be permanent internal change. Steve de Shazer (1985) nailed it when he offered that the attitude of the therapist should be to lead from one step behind.

The lesson learned is that we need to really listen to our clients and hear their knowledge and wisdom. Clients are our learning lab and there is no "one size fits all." Every family is unique and has its own unique culture. We need to learn more about the client sitting in front of us than merely an intake laundry list of history and goals. We need to learn about each client's problem-solving abilities and their culture of problem solving in order to be thorough and efficient in facilitating the change they seek. What works for each client and what needs to happen in order to unleash the power of "exceptions to the problem" can be elusive for the client. A skilled therapist who employs listening skills, neurolinguistic language, and strength-based, client-need-driven processes can help the client identify and embrace the keys to attaining desired change. Therapists will be the initiators of the process; but change—and thus the credit for change—will belong to the client.

Engaging and building a therapeutic alliance with a reluctant client who is mandated to treatment or who has been coerced to attend therapy can be achieved once we thoroughly understand that client's agenda and how they define the problem. There are tools and processes that—when individualized to be congruent with the features of the client's family, culture, strengths, and problem-solving history—will ultimately work to enhance outcomes for even the most reluctant clients who enter therapy as hopeless or impossible. Clients who were once labeled as resistant or difficult can achieve authentic, meaningful change, and can thrive. Too often, therapy is tainted from the start because the client's thinking and behaviors have been "pathologized," they are pressured into compliance, and the therapist's misperceptions thwart opportunities for positive attitudinal and behavioral change.

We can be effective with rich or poor; with those who are products of intact families or foster placement by social welfare agencies; with mandated or voluntary clients; with clients who have substance use disorders or behavioral disorders; with those in the justice system or law-abiding citizens; with persons diagnosed as having mood disorders or personality disorders; with elderly, middle-aged, or younger clients; or with individuals, couples, and families identifying with any gender, religion, diversity, or culture. The reasons behind the referral, modality, and life circumstances or diagnosis matter less than the therapeutic atmosphere and relationship we facilitate, and our willingness and ability to learn from the client "what works" for them. Keep in mind that for the most part, my clients—who we will be meeting throughout this book—did not realize how strong and resourceful they were at the time they entered therapy.

I am thrilled to share case examples, expressed as stories, that feature clients who found the courage and resolve to overcome despair and take risks. The case examples demonstrate how the character and resolve of clients will surface when they are treated as competent to identify solutions and solve their own problems. Client stories and interventions—some of which were originally presented as part of continuing education workshops over more than three decades—are illustrated throughout. Client anonymity was respected then and likewise is respected throughout this book. Individual clients and families are non-identifiable: details such as names, family composition, gender, employment, and some client history may have been masked, modified, or combined among clients with similar circumstances and outcomes to ensure confidentiality and privacy.

Featured case studies presented as client stories include the following:

- Linda did not know that she had everything she needed, and therapy got in her way.
- Cody, a Highway Patrol sergeant, was obsessed with the definition of change and if real change even existed.
- Arguing between Vicki and her mother exhausted their first therapist.
- Sarah feared she was no better than her mother.
- Johnny's addiction led him to believe that he was doomed to fail.
- Ten-year-old Billy suffered from bellyaches, but doctors could not find a physical cause.
- Tom's mother could not impact her teenage son's behavior and choices until she figured out how to bribe him.
- Kathy suffered panic attacks at work and was about to lose her job.
- A young single mother was going to be denied reunification with her children even though she had completed a court-ordered case plan and shown herself to be fit as a parent.
- Angie insisted that life should be enjoyable despite her history of trauma and depression.

- Eleven-year-old Terry in foster care wanted to overcome his past and be noticed for his good efforts.
- Teen Ashley was ready to sacrifice her own wellbeing and future in order to rescue her younger brother and fix her family.
- Lacy, a high-context communicator from Appalachia, was misunderstood and misdiagnosed.
- The dissonance for parents from the Philippines between their culture and the needs of their children exposed them to legal jeopardy.
- Adolescent Anna made a decision she regretted and needed a way to "save face" and participate in therapy with her family.
- A culture of multigenerational poverty put good parents at risk of losing custody of their children to Child Welfare.
- Mattie and her children were persecuted over their history, zip code, and culture.
- The Jones family were open to "doing something different," but therapist Jack was reluctant to assign a task.
- Ann and Tom were desperate to restore happiness and fun to their marriage.
- Sixteen-year-old Beth had run away from home 15 times and her stepfather was ready to leave her mother.
- Michelle needed to get back on track and somehow convince her husband to attend couples counseling.
- Bret was grieving his deceased wife and feeling desperate.
- Cathy needed her husband, Richard, to resolve his conflicts with her mother.

This book is in large part about the bumps and triumphs we encounter when we work with human beings for the greater good. I am grateful to the 1,000-plus clients and client families who trusted me with their secrets and vulnerabilities. I learned much from them about engaging and understanding people and families. Eventually, I learned how to really listen, hear, and be more receptive to the client's message, acknowledging their wisdom and strengths, and eliciting their solutions. Solution therapists know that when we engage clients in a collaborative process, therapy is more enjoyable and rewarding for both the therapist and the client. You will notice that those clients who began therapy in crisis, with despair and hesitancy, were eventually able to engage and participate in the language and tasks with lightheartedness and even humor.

It will be clear that using the client's language in defining the problem, and tapping into their personal strengths, history of problem solving, exceptions to the problem, and family culture, are important in creating a truly successful outcome. Any *tour de force* the reader finds in this book must be credited to clients and their persistence in finding solutions and improving the experience of life for themselves and their families. They were truly exceptional and heroic. My education, training, and clinical experiences may have been the metaphorical toolbox, but my clients were the ones who guided me in how and when to use the tools, if at all.

In reading this book, you will clearly see that in pursuit of better outcomes, I have evolved into a client-need-driven therapist. My overall objective is to facilitate a collaborative process as clients identify what they want in their own words, and then, as indicated, introduce clinical tools, strategies, and processes that will help them accomplish those goals. Carefully observing what is working or not working during therapy, I make whatever changes in my approach might be congruent with the client's preferred change processes. The outcomes the client wants are what matters. Decades of seeing client families in their community, training and supervising other clinicians, working with community treatment centers and agencies, and clinically managing research on solution-focused brief therapy (SFBT) with populations who have challenging issues afforded me invaluable feedback on what works.

In Chapter 1, I touch on my educational experiences, internships, training, and clinical work over five decades, including the impact of a new, distinct body of knowledge on my thinking and interventions with clients. Over decades of clinical work, I came to discern and refine the tools and methods compatible with SFBT that help to achieve successful outcomes for clients who do not want to be there, do not want therapy, do not believe they have a problem, and perhaps initially see you—their therapist—as unhelpful or even hurtful. Learning is enriched when knowledge builds on knowledge, so the next chapter also briefly discusses the evolution of the mental health field and clinical practice, including the impact of the new age founders, the birth of constructivist thinking, and the advances in engagement and solution therapy processes. I invite you to share that journey with me.

Reference

de Shazer, S. (1985) *Keys to Solution in Brief Therapy*. New York: W. W. Norton.

1   A Little About My Early Influences
Student of the Peace Corps Generation

More than 45 years ago, I entered the practice of psychotherapy with passion, optimism, and confidence. My expectation—albeit naïve—was that I would be the "expert" with the answers that would make a significant difference in the lives of my clients, whether individuals, couples, or families. The years of education and supervised internships that were so critical in obtaining licensure were behind me. My hope was that my passion, caring, and expertise in a variety of clinical approaches would be the impetus for me to be a trailblazer, leading to the birth of new interventions and methods.

As a graduate student, I can recall how I welled up with emotion as I daydreamed of future clients making life changes as a result of our work together. My generation was the Peace Corps generation—the generation of doing for others to make a positive difference. We were the healers, the fixers of the ills in the world, willing to put our physical safety on the line for civil rights and world peace. I was determined to be the best clinician possible, a healer for individuals and families. The "helping all of mankind" instinct was part of my makeup for as long as I can remember. It was as early as in the fifth grade that I made the decision to be a family therapist.

Psychology students in the 1960s were often educated first in psychodynamics. As a result, we were initially influenced in the direction of problem-focused, pathological thinking, and with the viewpoint that the clinician was the expert or "doctor." Client deficits were the focus of the intervention. Later, we were introduced to therapies from the humanistic school of thought, which looked at client strengths and competencies. Almost concurrently, we were taught about the new and older behavioral theories. The philosophical divide between Freudian, humanistic, and behavioral thinking was fervently expressed by professors invested in one or the other. Depending on which professor was your advisor or what school you were attending, it was common for individuals to be

DOI: 10.4324/9781003397380-1

strongly positioned in one of those philosophical camps—if not a new age "Freudian," you were a humanist or behaviorist—and spirited disagreements with those of the other persuasions were commonly heard in the classrooms and hallways of the campus buildings.

In the classroom, we were inculcated in the traditions and concepts of Freud, Skinner, Jung, Adler, Frankl, Rogers, Erik Erikson, and Maslow. Frankl's ideas (Frankl 1959) provoked thought about a "sense of purpose in life" or a "search for meaning," which resonated with a 20-year-old student trying to envision his future. Carl Rogers' beliefs (Rogers 1961) in client competency and empowerment fit well with the optimism and "power to the people" thinking of the time. I can attribute Rogers' ideas to the seed that eventually evolved into the development of good listening skills and respect for clients' ideas and competency; although others after him, such as Milton Erickson, were impactful with colorful stories in the modern client-centered movement (Zeig 1980). I also came to realize around that time that just the act of making an appointment and showing up takes courage and determination, and needs to be acknowledged for each client.

One-Way Mirror Work and Classroom Narratives for Learning and Feedback

Perhaps now a lost art, one-way mirror work was more than a skill-building tool. Reciprocal mirrors appear reflective on one side and transparent on the other. Being on a team that allowed us to watch when others worked with a client, and then give feedback, was empowering. If you were getting off track or missed an opportunity during a session, the team would ring a bell or buzzer, meaning that you were to take a break from the client and go behind the mirror to consult. Knowing that your team was watching and there to support you in constructive ways gave you the confidence to facilitate a session without fear of getting stuck or doing harm. It also provided the opportunity to try out what you had learned in classes, books, and roleplay. And although you might be a little nervous, having peers to interact with and sharing a few laughable moments went a long way to lift the tension or even make it fun. A colleague of mine had one of those interesting, laughable experiences during his initial "behind the mirror" experience.

The team suggested that he begin with a technique called "reflective listening"—a method for communicating to clients that you have heard and understand them. It involves merely repeating what the client has told you, using the client's words. A practitioner would hear: "Things have been very hard on me and my wife lately, so I decided to come here." The feedback would be phrased something like: "So you are saying that things have been very hard on you and your wife lately, and that is why you decided to come here." Essentially, the client's actual words are repeated, not the therapist's words or an interpretation of the client's words.

So, on that particular day, I observed from behind the mirror while my colleague was attempting his first counseling session with an actual client. The team had prepped him by repeating, "Begin with reflective listening." He sat down, introduced himself, and asked the client why he had decided to come to therapy. The client responded, "I'm here because my wife said that she was going to leave me if I didn't get help, and I don't even know what I did." My colleague hesitated for a moment, and then nervously replied, "I see. So, you're here because your wife said that she was going to leave you if you didn't get help, and you don't even know what you did." The client responded with, "I am so glad that you understand. I have the right therapist." My colleague continued to use reflective listening and after a couple of minutes, the bell rang. Behind the mirror with the team, my colleague's hands were shaking, and we all laughed as he said, "I can't believe that really worked!" He was awestruck by the simplicity and power of listening and merely reflecting back the words of the client to demonstrate understanding. A simple idea, but a powerful tool to validate, engage, and learn from our clients.

In the classroom, the most effective professors did not limit instruction to straightforward lectures about theories and concepts. Storytelling and vivid examples captured my attention and interest. Psychology became a bit more intriguing, and somewhat fascinating, when Gestalt therapy (Perls 1971) was introduced to us. Perls' concepts—referred to as "mystic" or "magical" by some students, and "outside the box" by others—provided us with concrete techniques to use in therapy sessions. We played around with the "empty chair" technique as a tool for the integration of inner conflict or to represent a person who was not present in therapy. Perls might have thought of our innovations as outliers! Later, during my academic internship, watching empty chair work from behind the mirror was more exciting than observing "talk therapy." In Chapter 5, I discuss an intervention using the empty chair to address panic attacks.

We might call their understanding of talk therapy crude, but the early founders of psychology truly did build the foundations on which our modern, evidence-based models and approaches would eventually stand. Yet it was not until late in graduate school that I was exposed to books and workshops bursting with newer, innovative methods, and advances in thinking and research that would revitalize the practice of effective psychotherapy and family systems thinking. Mental health work was evolving into a more friendly, creative, client-centered, and effective treatment profession. Interventions and outcomes with individuals, couples, and families benefited from new ideas and methods developed out of research on family systems, family dynamics, structural family assessment, client strengths, resilience, communication, addiction, behavior, culture, solution therapy, and how to differentiate between temporary change and genuine internal change.

The Impact of Cutting-Edge Research from the 1960s to the 1990s

I was fortunate that the advances in family therapy and client-centered solution work that began in the late 1960s continued to snowball throughout my years in private practice. Significant to my early professional development were several new influences, such as the Mental Research Institute (MRI), the Brief Family Therapy Center (BFTC), the Child Guidance Clinic in Philadelphia, and later Sal Minuchin's training and consultation Institute for Family Studies in New York City. A new, distinct body of knowledge was contributing to improved outcomes that required fewer sessions and featured authentic, lasting change. I refer to the pioneers responsible for this distinct body of knowledge as the "new age founders."

At the MRI, brilliant thinkers and clinicians with diverse backgrounds were looking at families as systems and clients as competent. The MRI was dedicated to scientific research based on new ways of looking at how people communicated and behaved, from which came revolutionary paradigms of change and innovations in treatment process. Their ideas relative to family dynamics, structure, rules, and roles were ground-breaking. "New age founders" and contributors at the MRI included the founder, Don Jackson, M.D.; John Weakland; Gregory Bateson; Richard Fisch, M.D.; Paul Watzlawick, Ph.D.; Murray Bowen, M.D.; Jay Haley, Ph.D.; Cloé Madanes, Ph.D.; Virginia Satir, MSW; Steve De Shazer, MSW; and briefly Insoo Kim Berg, MSSW, among others. de Shazer and Berg founded the BFTC, where they trained many young clinicians who went on to develop client-need-driven solution ideas. I was fortunate to have interacted with most of them and had the honor of participating in live trainings with several of them.

At the BFTC, the evolution of powerful new clinical practices resulted in processes to take clients into the future, with hope and the beginning of desired change starting now, rather than focusing on the past or even the present. Solution-focused brief therapy (SFBT) was developed through an iterative approach, which involves live observation with real clients to determine the words, questions, processes, and tasks that worked to achieve desired change, while removing features that did not contribute to good outcomes. SFBT is an evidence-based and practice-based evidence therapy, and a popular choice for therapists worldwide.

There were other innovative pioneers and researchers who were not directly affiliated with the MRI or the BFTC, such as Milton Erickson,

M.D. and Sal Minuchin, M.D.; as well as several Italian family psychiatrists—notably Maurizio Andolfi, M.D. and Luigi Boscolo, M.D.—whose insights and creativity added greatly to new understandings about mental illness and family dynamics. Their ideas and methods took us beyond the pathological, hopeless thinking about mental illness, including schizophrenia.

Books and papers written by the new age founders were popular among many therapists around the time I entered private practice, promoting ideas such as paying attention to what worked and what clients were telling clinicians, rather than doing the same thing repeatedly and then blaming the client if things did not work out well. Concepts around pathology and dysfunction were challenged, and many advances in the mental health field resulted. Ideas about the impact of family system dynamics in conjunction with working from client strengths and problem-solving skills were a departure from traditional methods. Their presence drew clinicians to professional conferences. State board licensing exams for clinicians tested knowledge of their names, ideas, and methods.

In Appendix A, I have listed some of the more influential new age founders with whom I have interacted. Their findings, concepts, and practice innovations are briefly summarized. I credit them with the advances that led to the highly successful client-need-driven interventions illustrated throughout this book. Research for decades has supported their ideas, and many of the "evidence-based" therapies are based at least partially on their concepts and theories.

Family Therapy Pioneers Challenged Mental Health Thinking and Practice

Differences or nonconformity in clients were commonly viewed as pathology in the mental health arena before the influence of the new age founders took hold. In 1952, the first official *Diagnostic and Statistical Manual of Mental Disorders* (DSM) classified homosexuality as a mental disorder. President Dwight D. Eisenhower banned homosexuals from working for the federal government. Conversion or reparative therapy was commonplace. In 1973, the American Psychiatric Association (APA) removed homosexuality as a mental health disorder from the *DSM*; and then 40 years later, in 2013, the APA made a statement that it did not believe that same-sex orientation should or needed to be changed, and that efforts to do so would represent a significant risk of harm. In 1975, the APA called on all mental health professionals to remove the stigma of mental illness associated with homosexuality; but it was not until 1993 that the National Association of Social Workers formally adopted a similar position. Homosexuality was not removed from *The ICD-10*,

International Classification of Diseases, the medical doctors' diagnostic manual, until 1990.

Thanks to the new age founders and their contemporaries, in addition to understanding family structure, family dynamics, and how family systems work, we now have effective strategies to help clients achieve resolution. Neurolinguistic research has significantly improved how we converse with clients and the words we use to formulate questions. Strategic thinking contributed to new ideas for tasks that helped promote change sooner, with fewer struggles for the therapist and client. Therapy evolved away from interventions that were directive toward client-centered and client-need-driven work. Listening to clients, understanding a client's definition of the problem, using the client's language, respecting the client's history and culture, and honoring what the client wants became new best practices for therapists. For the most part, the new age founders' names have been forgotten; but their groundbreaking ideas and methods are alive in our modern-day interventions and thinking about clients and families.

Initially, when I began work in private practice, I did not fully understand the power of strength-based, client-need-driven therapies. There were a few outstanding new age family therapists who offered "hands-on" workshops and attending those helped put me on the road to becoming a more complete "agent of change." In the 1980s, I was fortunate to become aware of SFBT and the research of Steve de Shazer and Insoo Kim Berg at the BFTC. I attended several of their trainings and worked at becoming skilled in SFBT concepts and processes. It was truly an honor to be an early disciple of their brilliant concepts and practices. Over the years, observing the change process with real clients in a variety of challenging settings, I have come to recognize the importance of a client's strengths and the need to rely on a client's expertise in order to achieve authentic, lasting change.

It is imperative for therapists to maintain an understanding of where they have been and the journey they have encountered before settling into their theoretical comfort zone. For many therapists, it is not easy to let go of the postures and models that were the foundation of our earliest education and training. Reflecting on both our early and later professional experiences can be invaluable for self-awareness and ultimately self-improvement in our clinical work. Client outcomes can serve as a mirror for us as we let go of the idea that the therapist is the expert and knows what is best for a client. As my career progressed and I came to more fully appreciate the client's right to autonomy and self-determination, I gained valuable insight into the pitfalls of "the clinician is the expert" therapy that too often "pathologizes" clients. (In Chapters 3 and 4 we discuss and differentiate between medical model and client-centered thinking.)

We will be reviewing some of the cornerstone practices to accomplish collaborative engagement and desired outcomes driven by our client. But first, let me share a story of regret that I have told in workshops and to interns over the years. Most, if not all of us have had those "I wish I had known then what I know now" moments and felt the accompanying pain and disappointment in ourselves. The intern in this story, well-meaning and otherwise competent, made an error because of his supervisor's mischaracterization of the "client." I could have made the same mistake early in my career before I knew better. Any of us could have made a similar mistake. In sharing this story, I explain that we all have had many high points in our careers, but this low point for that intern could haunt him for life. It checks all the boxes to describe a failed intervention: "Wrong therapist, wrong time, wrong circumstances, wrong issue."

Who Is Really the Client?

This was an unfortunate experience that can serve as an important lesson for all of us. An intern supervisor had asked one of his interns to complete a clinical assessment and intervene with a female offender in the city jail. When the intern arrived, the correctional sergeant and one of his fellow officers told him that they were concerned about the inmate's erratic behavior and angry mood. Let's call the inmate Reesha. Reesha was currently on parole from the state prison and had a long history of incarceration. Her arrest the evening before was for soliciting prostitution and attempting to rob her "John." She had been awake all night in her jail cell, yelling and screaming. None of the other inmates were able to sleep and staff were notably stressed.

The officer handed the intern a file that contained several years of psychological and medical histories, and recent notes from officers during the swing and graveyard shifts. Two of the officers had attached statements of concern from several inmates, who were familiar with some details of Reesha's history. One officer, who had been a correctional officer at the state prison when Reesha was an inmate there, wrote that she had been a victim of childhood physical and sexual abuse at the hands of her father. He concluded that the abuse from her father was the reason for Reesha's lifestyle as a prostitute who robbed "Johns." The statements from other inmates detailed concerns about Reesha being a victim of abuse and needing to deal with her history.

The intern was also given a file that was submitted by Reesha's parole officer. It contained years of documentation from the women's prison, including psychological and medical records, reports from correctional classification counselors, correctional officers, and parole officers. There were also copies of background forms, a life history, an old Minnesota

Multiphasic Personality Inventory, and parole documents that had been recently completed by Reesha. Essentially, the intern had ten years of behavioral testing, clinical documentation, and incident reports on a 28-year-old woman.

During a shift change that occurred shortly after his arrival, the intern was asked to wait in an office, which allowed him more than 20 minutes to read through the files. Once back in the confinement area, one of the correctional officers suggested that he talk with an inmate trustee who was working as an office janitor. The inmate knew Reesha from both prison and the streets. The intern spent about five minutes with her and received what sounded like a very objective history, certainly consistent with the psychological and medical history, officers' statements, inmate statements, and chronology that he had just read in the files.

The intern's stomach churned as he heard about and reflected on the abuse and trauma Reesha had experienced throughout her childhood, and how the correctional system had aggravated the problem by re-traumatizing her instead of providing services that might have initiated a process for emotional healing. He felt fortunate to have been given some insight into Reesha's history and the issues that must have been burdening her. His heart went out to her, and he was determined to be the one person who made a difference. To be certain of his role and clarify some of his thoughts, he called his supervisor just before meeting with Reesha. Hearing his compassion for Reesha, his supervisor cautioned, "I know it's hard to process everything that happened to her; but remember that you are there at the request of the jail. Their staff have to put up with her behavior. They are your clients."

Who was the client? Reesha? The staff at the jail? Both? Here's the rest of the story …

The intern then formulated a plan and took a low-key approach as he introduced himself and told Reesha that he was there to see if he could be helpful. Completing paperwork that included an informed consent went smoothly. Reesha was quiet and calm with him, so he decided to use the available time to address what might be the "root cause" of her problems in order to achieve a quick resolution. Thinking that he was engaging her in a way that demonstrated concern, he asked, "Who hurt you as a child?" Reesha stood up and yelled, "My father built seven churches!" She then folded her arms and refused to talk to him. Her screaming resumed, and she had to be restrained. Thereafter, she refused to cooperate with other clinicians while in jail.

The intern was stunned and felt guilty. Lesson learned, perhaps; but Reesha was re-traumatized and had to be put on suicide watch. The intern thought he knew enough about Reesha to understand how to approach her, but obviously he did not. What he did accomplish was to close off any chance of building a trust relationship with her. The contents of the files had addressed the concerns about Reesha's history and behaviors from previous clinicians and correctional staff. No one had asked Reesha what she needed, or offered to be an advocate or ombudsman if she needed an ally. There were no indications that even one of the clinicians had attempted to develop a collaborative therapeutic alliance with her. As can too often be the case, others were more invested in solving their problem—Reesha's disruption—than sincerely addressing Reesha's needs.

In Chapter 3 we discuss a client's "agenda"—in other words, "what the client really wants." The intern in this story had felt pressure to address the agenda of the jail staff. He never elicited the agenda of inmate Reesha, so he was unable to address it. Her agenda is not going to be the product of what is in a file or what the referral source says. Much of this book addresses differing agendas and keeping a pulse on the needs of the client in front of you. It is true that if you work for an agency or under a grant, you may have obligations and a degree of loyalty to them; but they are not your client in the same sense as someone with whom you have a clinical relationship. We may also have a connection to the referral source—the court, an agency, a relative, society in general—and some obligation to report to them; but they are not our primary client.

Best practice requires interventions to allow our clients to teach us about themselves. How a client defines the problem, their culture, family, strengths, and goals will define pieces of our intervention. Experience over the years, working with very wise colleagues, has taught me that we need to get a history directly from the client, using the client's words, before we can figure out how to effectively engage even those clients who say they "don't want therapy." The truth is, most of us are inclined to invent parts of our reality; but what matters is that we give priority to helping a client facilitate desired changes rather than trying to "correct the record." When we gather information from other sources, we can be vulnerable to making judgments and drawing conclusions that will make us ineffective and unwelcome. Listening to clients from a "one-down position" is likely the best way to determine what they are invested in and what will work for them.

A Career Featuring a Diversity of Clients and Settings

In my professional career, I have had the opportunity to work and learn in a variety of settings. My experience has included working as a therapist in private practice, medical facilities, community treatment centers, child welfare agencies, juvenile justice, and adult corrections, including prisons. Perhaps the most impactful learning experience I encountered occurred when I was hired as the regional research site supervisor and clinical manager for a national research and demonstration project on intensive in-home therapy with low-resource, high-risk families in the child welfare and juvenile justice systems. It was my early training with Insoo Kim Berg years before that opened the door to this opportunity.

In the 1990s, several esteemed mental health professionals—including Insoo Kim Berg (Berg 1994) —became interested in working with families in the child welfare system. Historically, clinical work with child welfare clients had not produced desired outcomes, and a number of protective services programs were reducing or diverting their funding for therapeutic interventions with families. The number of children placed into foster care was overwhelming the system. Insoo began clinical research with child welfare populations and was able to demonstrate promising results using SFBT. Several jurisdictions applied for federal grants targeted at research on SFBT with families at imminent risk of having their children removed from the family home and placed into foster care. Clientele in the study featured families coerced into therapy who were not invested in treatment and did not trust the "system." As an early disciple of SFBT, in December 1994, I was selected as the regional research site supervisor and clinical manager for one of those programs.

We worked with culturally diverse families; multigenerational poverty; children in the juvenile justice system; middle-class families; children and families with disabilities; victims of trauma; family members with an arrest history; parents with addictions to substances and mental health issues; families in rural settings and in inner cities; and those impacted by racism. Prior to our research, many of the client families were considered "hopeless" cases. Our clinicians, supported by the work of researchers and using SFBT, were able to accomplish effective strategies for collaborative engagement with coerced and court-ordered clients who were reluctant to participate in family therapy. The SFBT process—coupled with structural family assessments, strategic tasking, neurolinguistic strategies, and other addendums—was effective in maintaining safety, improving family functioning, and preserving families for children.

In addition to learning a great deal about high-risk, low-resource client families during the demonstration project and clinical research at Intensive Family Services (IFS), I came to appreciate the difficulties posed by poverty and the challenges faced by people of color regardless of their cooperation and willingness to follow directives and court orders required to preserve their family. We learned about the resilience and strength of even the most disadvantaged client families facing significant challenges, and what really works to help unleash their power and potential. Once I understood how to engage clients with this extraordinary approach, I knew that any situation or issue had the potential to be manageable. (Chapter 11 delves into some of the unique experiences and lessons learned from client families in the child welfare population.)

Following my tenure as regional research site supervisor and clinical manager for IFS, I continued in private practice. Applying what we learned at IFS, I focused on accepting referrals of "impossible" clients from other providers, managed care insurance companies, and employee assistance programs; contracted to provide clinical services, clinical supervision, and training for treatment centers and government-funded programs; consulted with therapists when they sought assistance with clients whom they found to be "difficult"; and developed and facilitated workshops for continuing education. I had been noticing that many clinicians who got "stuck" when their clinical model processes were not working religiously continued with the same structured questions and sequences instead of securing an opportunity for collaborative engagement or offering a task to achieve the outcome the client said they wanted. I knew then that I would have to write this book.

This book is a product of my direct clinical experience; research site supervision at IFS; consultation with agencies and treatment centers; and interaction with supervisors, interns, and clinicians. Woven throughout are case studies which present the stories of courageous clients who overcame difficult circumstances, and during their journey affirmed that attending to the client's definition of the problem, philosophy of change, culture, family history, and "what they really want" cements the foundation on which to build an individualized clinical process that really works. SFBT theory and methods are meaningfully sequenced throughout each chapter, along with supplemental collaborative processes and innovative tools that empower and motivate even the most reluctant clients to engage and identify solutions that fit for them. The supplemental client-need-driven strategies and tools fit seamlessly with SFBT process work.

The next chapter discusses one of the transformational learning points in my career, just prior to attending trainings and workshops with Insoo Kim Berg and Steve de Shazer.

References

Berg, I. K. (1994). *Family Based Services: A Solution-Focused Approach.* New York: Norton

Frankl, V. (1959). *Man's Search for Meaning.* Boston: Beacon Press.

Perls, F. D. (1971). *Gestalt Therapy Verbatim.* London: Bantam Press

Rogers, C. (1961). *On Becoming a Person.* New York: Houghton Mifflin Company.

Zeig, J.K. (ed.) (1980). *A Teaching Seminar with Milton H. Erickson, M.D.* New York: Brunner/Mazel.

2 The Problem-Solving Process
We Often See Clients at Their Worst

One of my early insights about the challenges faced by clients and therapists came from a client, Linda, who made an appointment with me to talk about overwhelm and stress in her routine. Her closest friend, who had recently had a positive experience attending therapy, suggested that Linda see a counselor because it would be the best way to get in touch with her feelings and goals, and stay the course.

Linda was an intelligent, serious, and well-spoken client who presented with complaints of intermittent sleep disruption and fatigue, along with one or two days a week of either overeating or loss of appetite. She shared that at one time she had high expectations that the decisions she had made about her career, marriage, and family would bring her happiness. A married career woman with two active elementary school-aged children for whom she was the primary caretaker, she had a stressful job, and a busy schedule.

Linda revealed that she had been thinking about and even rehearsing what she would say in therapy for weeks, so she finally decided it was time to make an appointment. During a standard intake session, I gathered information about medical, social, psychological, and family history, and inquired about goals in therapy. From her disclosure, and observation during the next several sessions, it appeared that her symptoms met the criteria for a diagnosis of dysthymia—a chronic mood disorder characterized by symptoms of mild to moderate depression.

Sitting somewhat awkwardly in a large, blue overstuffed chair in my office, she would take out a list of her complaints and go through each one at the start of our sessions. I asked questions to clarify, and then demonstrated understanding and empathy, employing a trove of client-centered methods to help enhance her self-awareness and self-understanding. We would discuss tasks that might help, and I would prescribe strategic "homework" in the hope that it might ameliorate her symptoms. Even when a task would seem to help lighten her stress, she would bring up new complications and challenges during the next appointment from a fresh list of concerns.

DOI: 10.4324/9781003397380-2

Nothing she brought up sounded like pathology, but she presented as overwhelmed and desperate for resolution.

Initially, Linda had hoped psychotherapy would be a solution for her feelings and the adjustment difficulties that she attributed to changes in her workplace. She also brought up concerns about meeting her children's needs and the stressors attributed to balancing work with the needs of her family. As we discussed the issues she raised, it was apparent that "peeling the layers of the onion" was helpful only in uncovering or increasing difficulties and sadness. Her list was always current, specific, and helpful in painting a picture of her unhappy thoughts and experiences from the previous week. I felt sympathetic toward her and her never-ending battles week after week.

One Saturday morning, I was sitting on the top level of the aluminum bleachers at a city soccer field. Linda was sitting about 50 feet to my right in the adjoining bleachers with a group of parents whom she apparently knew. Her son was playing for one of the teams. She was laughing, cheering, talking to her friends, and generally presenting as happy—even elated—as she rooted for her son's team and interacted with her friends. I observed her for more than an hour that day, and she did not acknowledge me. Generally, in consideration of confidentiality and privacy, I am careful to avoid contact with my clients in public.

By coincidence, the next day I was in a supermarket to pick up a few items and I heard what sounded like Linda's voice. Sure enough, an aisle over, she was talking to a couple as she selected items for her grocery cart. Linda was expressive and bubbly, and she spoke proudly about her children's accomplishments and a weekend getaway that she, her husband, and her sister and brother-in-law had enjoyed some weeks previously. I stayed an aisle from her and continued to listen, learning that she was picking up last-minute items for her daughter's birthday party later that afternoon. Could this be the same Linda who I had been seeing in counseling sessions?

The next week, Linda came to her therapy session with a list of issues and complaints, but no mention of soccer, a birthday party, or the weekend getaway. Then I had an epiphany so unnerving that I felt my heart in my throat: Linda's problems were at least partially my fault, and my services were making her condition worse rather than better. I questioned her in detail about her week and her list of complaints, admitting that I had seen her at soccer and in the grocery store. What she shared with me forever changed how I would do therapy!

I learned that a few days before our sessions, Linda would consciously begin to think about the things that concerned her or caused her to feel unhappy. She would then begin to compile a written list of what she "needed" to discuss with me. Linda explained that her impression about getting the most out of therapy meant that she was supposed to prepare to talk about problems. Her focus for those few days before our appointment was on stressors, unfulfilled dreams, disappointments, and challenges in her life. She worked hard to develop a problem list that included anything even remotely negative about her feelings, thoughts, and interactions. Symptoms of sadness, sleep disruption, appetite issues, and fatigue would manifest and then increase over the days just prior to our session. Linda would then present with a depressed mood and often in an awkward, somewhat detached manner.

Coincidentally, just prior to our next appointment, I attended a workshop facilitated by Insoo Kim Berg and Steve De Shazer on solution-focused brief therapy (SFBT) and research they had completed. At the time of setting appointments with clients, they would ask about the presenting problem and then direct clients to bring to the first appointment a list of the things that they were happy about and did not want to change (de Shazer 1985, p. 137). What Insoo and Steve discovered was stunning: most clients reported that the presenting problem was no longer an issue for them when they arrived for the first session. There was also a discussion in the group that when people are overwhelmed by life's circumstances, they lose sight of their problem-solving strengths. Now I had a better understanding of what I needed to explore with Linda, and why I had been stuck.

The following week, I discussed a different kind of task with her. "Linda, think about the blessings in your life—those things that you are happy about and want to continue. Think about and make a list of the things you do not want to change," I suggested. I explained to her that in future sessions, as an experiment, we would begin with those things that she was happy about, and then we could talk about her problems. "This could give me a more complete picture of how to be helpful," I explained. Linda cheerfully committed to think about and write down those things that she did not want to change during the week just prior to our meetings, and to begin each session by reviewing that list with me. She agreed to allocate half the session to talk about things that were not problems, and half to talk about problems.

Our next appointment began with a discussion of the things on the list that were going well, which she liked and did not want to change. After Linda had shared the items on what she called her "don't want to change list," she responded to clarifying questions with more detail about her children, family, and the fulfilling events of the week. I then asked Linda about her problem list. It was clear to both of us that her reading of the problem list lacked the usual emphasis, and details in her follow-up comments were limited or absent. For the remainder of the session, she initiated a discussion that primarily focused on how well her children were doing in school and how proud she was of them. I could see and hear a strong and positive tone and mood that reminded me more of the Linda I had overheard at the soccer field and in the grocery store.

By the next session, two weeks later, Linda reported that difficulties with sadness, sleep, appetite, and fatigue had mostly resolved. She had an extensive list of the happy, "don't want to change" items, which she enthusiastically read and discussed. Her mood was elated, and she laughed several times. After Linda had finished answering a few clarifying questions and talking about plans for a family vacation during the next school break, the session was almost half over. She indicated that it was difficult for her to create a list of negative things after writing down the positives. What came to mind, Linda shared, were two minor incidents that had not gone as well as she had intended. After presenting the details, she concluded that those incidents were just annoying but normal family stuff.

Following one additional session in which Linda reported no problems of any significance, we changed the frequency of therapy appointments to a few follow-ups and then "as needed." We met four times over the next six months, and at each meeting Linda reported that her mood and outlook were positive. On a 0-10 scale, she rated her family life and work life as 9 or 10 during each subsequent session. Linda responded well to validation and discussion of her strengths and accomplishments. I transitioned with her into question sequences that took her into the future to look at goals and how she was going to accomplish them. She thrived!

One feature of living in a moderately sized suburban community with a storied downtown is that you will regularly run into people that you know. I would see Linda several times a year at various events around town, in restaurants, or shopping. She clearly presented as upbeat and energetic. At times she has acknowledged me and bragged about her children's successes. She is a proud mom! Linda has referred several clients to me and told each one that they did not have to be "down in the dumps" to benefit from therapy.

My experience with Linda taught me that as therapists, we can inadvertently make the quality of life worse for our clients by creating an atmosphere that addresses problems without a balance. I saw Linda as a "troubled" person who was overwhelmed by life and family issues. I did not fully understand that often we see clients at their worst; and we can miss recognizing a client's strengths, achievements, and triumphs because they often present with a focus on problems or disappointments. Therapists can be vulnerable to mistaking intent and the desire for self-improvement or support as being overwhelmed or having a disorder. Until I recognized that the problem was the approach I was using, I was unable to help Linda find resolution. I needed to do something different, so I made changes in my work with Linda and in my approach with future clients.

Problem talk is important for understanding and hearing the client's definition of the problem; but there needs to be an early transition where we elicit goals, exceptions, and solutions. Unless a client is in crisis, it can be powerful to switch gears during a client history and cultural assessment. Intake should include a process to learn about strengths and successes, including problem solving history and being cognizant to hear the client's language and philosophy of change—in other words, how change happens for that client. SFBT provides evidence-based processes including neurolinguistic language and question sequences that empower clients to acknowledge but look beyond their presenting problem. Clients usually benefit from cheerleading. My feedback is heavy with compliments that reflect a client's strengths, coping skills, and successes. Whenever practical, any future session begins with a discussion of, "What's better?"

Problem-Solving History Process

An insightful trainer once said to me, "If 'telling' a client what to do really worked, our prisons would be empty." Although clients often look to their mental health clinician for answers, it is the clients themselves who have the knowledge and wisdom to overcome their challenges. Client strength-based thinking—relying on the client as the expert—will result more often in solutions that work, and thus in better outcomes. We need to empower clients—through our questions, feedback, and compliments—to find their answers and believe in their personal power to solve problems. I have come to understand that we need to put clients in charge of finding their solutions by modeling the SFBT "problem-solving history process." If we try to be the experts, what happens may look like real change, but relapse or recidivism will often follow.

What I refer to as the "problem-solving history process" is a way of thinking, of processing, of finding answers and solutions based on a client's experience with similar circumstances. It is also a tool for empowerment that can lead to the development of resilience and self-sufficiency. Therapists can use it with clients; but in fact, most anyone can use it as part of self-talk. Once this thinking is internalized, it can be applied to any challenges faced in the future. Therapists can learn "what works" for a client by listening to their insights and solutions.

Here are two examples of the problem-solving history process that can uncover and enhance a client's skills at problem solving:

- "When have you encountered a problem—maybe similar to this one—that you were able to resolve?"

- "How did you do that?"
- "What helped?"
- "Who was helpful?"

Then, as feedback, talk about and compliment successes and strengths that came from that discussion. Let your client know that you are impressed by their efforts and insights. Elicit more ideas as you give feedback. And then ask:

- "Knowing what you know from that experience, what might you do now and in the future...?"
- "What needs to happen to achieve [the desired outcome that would replace the problem]"?
- "How have you done some of that in the past?"
- "What part of this are you beginning to do now? (Even a little bit?)"
- "What needs to happen for you to do more of it?"
- "What will be different when that happens?"
- "What is already different because you have started to move in that direction?"
- "Who will notice first that it has happened—that you have done it?"
- "How will you know when it has happened—what will you begin to notice is different?"

Client strength-based thinking provides many opportunities for both therapist and client. It is not merely calling our client competent and asking for exceptions and solutions. Client-centered and client-need-driven approaches are based on a way of thinking and viewing that is different than some of the more traditional therapeutic methods. A collaborative relationship with the client positioned as the "expert" can lead to change dynamics that are powerful and lasting. Clients will acquire and internalize tools that they can access to address and resolve future difficulties. Referencing an old adage, it is about teaching a client to fish rather than giving the client a fish. Which type of therapist do you want to be?

Understanding Client Recidivism and the Dynamics of Change

Client recidivism is frustrating for clients and professionals. Therapists will tell you that they have a fair number of clients who have responded well in therapy, only to return for additional help after "successful" discharge. Some of those clients have reverted to the "old" behaviors that brought them to therapy, while others have regressed into more severe patterns with serious consequences. The clinical interaction and therapeutic approach used with clients are prime determinants of the strength and permanence of change. Understanding the various "types" of change, and knowing the characteristics of each, can be insightful for clinicians.

In the late 1980s, a discussion with a Highway Patrol sergeant helped me to conceptualize and better explain the change experience. Cody sought me out in order to address issues that had manifested over 20 years of traffic enforcement and accident investigation. He was frustrated with citizens who did not heed safety protocols and speed limits, and said he could not understand why—in spite of unpleasant or even deadly consequences—many drivers did not buckle their seatbelts. The hairs on the back of my neck stood up when he said, "I've seen many deaths on the highway, but never have I had to unbuckle a corpse from a seatbelt."

Cody shared stories of chronic speeders and distracted drivers:

> I try to educate them a little when I give a warning or ticket, but my words and common sense don't seem to matter. The lucky ones don't crash and die but they get tickets with fines that they can't afford, and I know their insurance rates must increase. Some lose their licenses and can't get to work unless they drive illegally. Often, I notice them on the road again during the next year—yes, I remember every car I ticket—and they drive safely for a while. But then at some point they are again shaving or putting on makeup while driving; and speeding, making unsafe lane changes, or not buckling up. It's as if all the words and consequences never mattered.

Cody told me a story about how the Highway Patrol developed a plan to more effectively use their newest "instant on" radar gun technology. Unbeknown at the time, he provided me with fodder to understand the dimensions of change. In workshops over the years, I have used metaphor and Cody's information to explain to clinicians the dynamics of compliance, first-order change, and second-order change. I have borrowed the terms "first-order change" and "second-order change" from a systems therapy concept used at the Mental Research Institute, which distinguishes between surface change versus permanent system change (Watzlawick P., Weakland J.H.& Fisch 1974, p.12). My presentation to the group of workshop attendees generally proceeds as follows:

Saul: How many of you have had a number of clients who have done really well in therapy, and you discharge them with high hopes; but then several months later, or in a year or two, they're back in therapy with similar problems?
[Everyone nods, says "yes," or indicates familiarity in some manner.]

Saul:	So, let me ask a seemingly unrelated question. How many of you exceed the speed limit regularly?
	[Just about everybody raises their hand.]
Saul:	Okay—where do you mostly speed?
	[Group identifies local highways/freeways such as I-580.]
Saul:	So, you are driving down I-580 and the speed limit is, what— 65 most of the way?
Group:	65 or 70.
Saul:	So how fast are you going?
Group:	75 ... /80 ... /85 ...
	[Consensus becomes 80.]
Saul:	Okay, you're driving 80 in a 65 zone, and you see a Highway Patrol cruiser parked on the shoulder. What do you do?
Group:	Slow down ... /Take my foot off the accelerator ... /I don't want to hit the brakes or he'll see the brake lights ...
Saul:	How fast are you going now?
Group:	The speed limit—65.
Saul:	For how long do you stay at 65?
Group:	Maybe until I can't see him in my rear-view mirror—like a mile, maybe less.
Saul:	That is called *compliance*. As long as you're being watched or monitored; or if you think your behavior is being noticed; or maybe you are close to getting caught; or if you want things to settle down for now, you act like and look like you've made a change in behavior. But it is merely *compliance*. Temporary, situational. Most of our clients are good at *compliance*.
	Law enforcement knows a lot about human behavior. They study it. I used to know a Highway Patrol sergeant. He told me a story about how they figured out the best way to set speed traps after they got the new "instant on" radar guns in the 1980s. Cody had some interesting information to share about speeders. Do you know the number one excuse drivers use when pulled over to try to get out of a speeding ticket?
	[Several guesses from group.]
Saul:	The number one excuse is, "Officer, I didn't realize that I was speeding. Sorry." The sergeant told me that they are not so interested in ticketing the occasional or accidental speeder who looks at the speedometer and says to themselves, "Oh my gosh, I'm going seven miles over the speed limit; I'd better slow down," as they are in ticketing the chronic speeder. So how do you tell the difference? Here's how: they park a cruiser on the shoulder of a highway. Drivers passing by check their speed and slow down if they're speeding. Then after a mile or so the

real speeders will speed up, when they think they're "in the clear." The Highway Patrol has chase cars a mile or two up the road with "instant on" radar guns. You're going 80. You get pulled over and say, "Officer, I didn't realize I was speeding." The officer knows everyone checked their speed a mile back, and that you're a liar and most likely a chronic speeder—so you get a ticket. Pretty smart, isn't it?

[Lots of squirming in seats and groans; it's obvious that at least several participants personally recognize this scenario.]

Saul: So, how do you drive now that you've gotten a ticket?

Group: Different ... /Better ... /Slower ... /At the speed limit or close to it ... /Carefully ...

[Almost everyone, if not everyone, indicates that they would now drive at the speed limit or very close to it.]

Saul: I see. You drive at the speed limit or very close to it—but for how long?

Group: Until it comes off my record ... /Until it doesn't affect my insurance anymore ... /For a short while ... /For a few months ... / For a year ... /It depends on how many points I have ...

[And similar answers.]

Saul: You've changed your driving habits. You want to drive at the speed limit for a while. You really have changed—but only temporarily, until something occurs or doesn't occur. You don't want a higher insurance premium, or to lose your license, or go to traffic school. You're waiting for it to be off your record or to be ticket free for a year. You've just described first-order change. It is temporary, external change that often looks like real change. Therapists and maybe some clients get fooled and think it's real change. We discharge our clients and then they're back in therapy or in trouble a year later. How many of you can relate to seeing this happen with clients?

[Almost everyone or everyone raises their hands.]

Saul: Let's say the governor calls you and says:

> *I've been told that you are a smart and reasonable person. I need your help. Our citizens need your help. We have a problem with chronic speeding. There are too many accidents— too many fatalities and serious injuries. There are also complaints about speed limits—too slow, too fast. I need someone to partner with me and head a committee to study all the speed limit information and make a decision about the proper speed limits on every road statewide. We would like you to select whomever you want: family, friends,*

professionals, co-workers, people you trust. We'll give you all the data about roads, accidents, safety information, physics of speed, weather, conditions—literally everything you need to know. We'll make physicists, highway engineers, and road, driving, and weather experts available to you. Consult with your committee, study the information, drive the roads, and think this through. You will be the expert. Complete your study and assign a speed limit to every road in the State, including highways and residential streets. It's up to you.

You accept the governor's request, select the committee, consult the experts, do the complete study, make the decisions, and submit your findings and recommendations. Every change in speed limits you have suggested is accepted and put in place by the governor. How are you going to drive in the future?

Group: At the speed limit … /Probably at the speed limit … /Not over the speed limit … /At about the speed limit … /I decided it, so I will follow it … /Maybe I'm annoyed at cars that are speeding …

[The consensus—with very few if any exceptions—is that they would drive at the speed limit.]

Saul: We've just described second-order change. It is internal change, real change. Lasting change. It is because this was a collaborative process that allowed you to be the expert. The exact "how to" was elicited from you, and you made the decision regarding what to change after considering the information. This is what we want to achieve with our clients. Real and lasting change comes from a process that involves respecting the client as the expert and eliciting client solutions, not telling the client what to do and how to do it. When you as the therapist provide the solutions, they are your solutions, not the client's.

In Appendix B, "Dynamics of Change," I have summarized and defined the three features of change.

Therapists are agents of change; but clients are experts on what change looks like and on the decision to change or not change—a clinical concept applied throughout *Clues: Investigating Solutions in Brief Therapy* (de Shazer 1988). We are impacting more than the client sitting in front of us. Future generations will be positively or negatively affected by the skill of a therapist to either create an environment for healthy change or get in the way. In Chapter 3, we explore the values and ideas that are the bones of client centeredness and client-need-driven process, and then look at how their application facilitates a process conducive to growth and second-order change.

References

de Shazer, S. (1985). *Keys to Solution in Brief Therapy*. New York: Norton.
de Shazer, S. (1988). *Clues: Investigating Solutions in Brief Therapy*. New York: Norton.
Watzlawick, P., Weakland, J. H. and Fisch, R. (1974). *Change: Principles of Problem Formation and Problem Resolution*. New York: Norton.

3   Lessons Learned

The Bones of Client Centeredness and Client-Need Driven Process

It was my good fortune to attend advanced workshops and seminars for continuing education, facilitated by those brilliant new age clinicians and researchers who understood the dynamics of the family and individual, and were able to define change and the process needed to get there on the family's terms. The pioneers of positive change processes had figured out how to use talk therapy to identify a client's strengths and history of successes, no matter how small; to understand each client's unique problem-solving skills; to empower and motivate clients toward the growth and change they wanted; and to then let the client be the expert in identifying and implementing solutions, rather than giving advice or telling the client what to do. Their workshops and seminars provided the new rules of the road for successful clinical work.

Good intentions, optimism, and positive energy will keep us fresh and committed to our clients. An open mind and the ability to maintain hope can help a therapist stay on track and facilitate successes with even clients who arrive with the most challenging issues. To reiterate, the client, not the professional, is the expert on their own life; and when solutions are properly elicited from the client, the outcomes are more likely to be attainable and lasting. My personal journey from "I am the professional expert" to "I can be helpful, but the client is the expert" involved substantive and sometimes unsettling insights. Compliance is easy for most clients, but is temporary; whereas real change—referred to in the previous chapter as "second-order change"—requires an internal process from the client. An authentic change process requires a therapist to learn how to be a catalyst for real change and not get in the way.

Eliciting Solutions and Trusting the Client's Strengths and Resourcefulness

The therapeutic alliance must be collaborative if it is to be effective. Eliciting solutions from the client enhances and fuels positive energy for change.

DOI: 10.4324/9781003397380-3

When a client owns the change, there is a greater investment in success. Hope, confidence, and willingness are built into the equation because the change is not merely an abstract concept from the clinician, but an expectation defined by the client in the client's own words. The therapist helps the client to refine the picture of change by asking questions that will further define the change in concrete, measurable behaviors. Those behaviors become the goals, which then can be further defined by small increments of change. Remarkably, therapists who understand the concept of small, incremental change will recognize change that is already beginning to happen and thus can "throw success in the client's face" even before the client is fully aware that progress has been achieved.

A key breakthrough in my understanding of how to help clients identify the change they want and achieve successful outcomes was the insight that therapeutic skill is about learning strategies that allow us to learn from our clients. When clients can teach us how to help them, we become more effective. Too often, therapists unwittingly block clients from taking the driver's seat in initiating and accomplishing change. Those who are "married" to a clinical model or directive approach may have an expectation that clients who do not respond are "resistant." Clinicians who use "cookie-cutter" approaches can find it challenging to let go of the "expert" moniker and consider client-need-driven strategies for engagement. Cookie-cutter methodology fails to address the beliefs and uniqueness of each individual client.

A "client-centered," "client-need-driven" approach employs interventions tailored to fit the specific individual. In order to be a receptive, skillful listener and allow clients to use their knowledge and expertise, own the change, and take control of their lives, we need to accept several premises about our clients and ourselves. We will discuss these premises and then look at how their application made it possible for a teenage girl, Vicki, and her mother to overcome a conflict that had consumed them for years.

Respect Clients as Experts in Their Domain

The starting point is to accept that clients are the experts in their domain and are competent and resourceful. We know that effective therapy results when there is collaboration between the client and the therapist. Collaboration requires an agreement between the client and clinician on goals and tasks. Without client participation and buy-in, it would not be possible to effectively work toward real, lasting solutions. The key to an effective change process is to first hear from clients how they define the problem and about times when they have had the problem under control. We can learn from our clients how solutions or partial solutions happen for them.

Prioritize Your Client's Agenda

Client "agendas" are at the core of client centeredness, engagement, and goal setting. A client's agenda can be defined as "what the client really wants." Identifying and prioritizing the client's agenda is what will make the client a customer for therapy. Too often, a client's agenda is not acknowledged, and even disregarded. The court's agenda, the referring agency's agenda, or the therapist's agenda might be different than the client's agenda. Unless we hear and acknowledge the client's agenda, the client will not be available or invested in authentic change. Before the therapeutic process can bear fruit, we need to discuss with our client and validate what they are invested in.

"Client-need driven" works better than "agency or program-need driven." In other words, avoid the pre-packaged agenda offered by an agency, program, or clinical model; and listen to the needs and goals of your client. Rather than imagining what you would want for yourself, or what makes sense to you for your client to pursue, listen and be accepting of the client's priorities first. Using yourself as the standard for "normal" is poor methodology if you are seeking client engagement and a good clinical result. If you can be helpful now from the client's point of view, there will opportunities to introduce, through eliciting, other issues that the client may need to address before treatment ends. Additional goals can be identified and then added later. For now, think of the client's agenda as the gold standard!

Court orders or a referral agency's requirements are not ignored. Someone else's agenda can be discussed with the client; but the client's agenda must take center stage. When there is, for example, a court order, we could inquire what our client is willing to do about it; but it may not be the client's priority or number one goal. Ideally there would be an opportunity to work on the client's agenda and the court order concurrently. We might acquire some insight by asking questions such as:

- "How will you know when you don't have to come here anymore?"
- "What needs to happen for you to say this time with me has been worthwhile?"
- "What do you think the judge/your wife/your social worker would say you need to do?"

Later, we will explore a series of more in-depth process questions that have been shown to be effective in validating and processing a client's agenda and goals.

Clients—especially mandated clients—will often tell you what they think you want to hear. Certainly, this is understandable because their primary agenda, for example, might be that they want to "get out of trouble" or "get their spouse off their back," and they may not think it will make a good impression to put it that way. We need to be respectful and not label a client as dishonest or resistant just because they are trying to protect themselves or their family, or because they are not invested in what somebody else thinks they need. We will discuss ideas around "resistance" later; but for now, it is crucial to make your client a customer by respecting and prioritizing their agenda, and to focus first on what parts of the agenda are changeable, not intractable. When we acknowledge and cheerlead small successes, and a mandated client sees that our services are worthwhile, more often than not it will be possible at some point to engage them around the reason for referral.

Attend to Your Client's Hierarchy of Needs

We too often lose perspective and miss a client's agenda because we do not consider or fully understand the impact of Maslow's "hierarchy of needs" on the client. Clinicians working in the juvenile justice and child welfare systems, as well as in private practice, acquire a keen awareness that a client's priorities, or agenda, will be greatly impacted by their circumstances and needs. For example, looking at a client's "case plan" or "court order," we might be addressing ways that the client can improve confidence and verbal skills in order to interview for a job; while the client may be worried about how they are going to feed their children today. In all cases, the client's hierarchy of needs will significantly affect their agenda, engagement in therapy, and completion of assigned tasks.

A Collaborative Therapeutic Relationship is the Primary Determinant of Success

A therapeutic atmosphere and a collaborative therapeutic relationship will be the primary determinants of a successful outcome. Client-centered therapists are skilled at employing Rogerian core conditions (Rogers 1961) such as respect, positive regard, genuineness, active listening, and empathy throughout the process. Research over the years has consistently validated the importance of relationship building and Rogerian principles of joining and engaging. There are complex factors working against collaborative engagement with mandated or coerced clients. Successful strategies are discussed and illustrated in future chapters.

The power differential between a therapist and client invariably can work against a trust relationship. Too often, therapists inadvertently become parents, cops, or prosecutors in the dialog and interaction. Respecting the client as the expert in their domain, and eliciting exceptions and solutions instead of "telling," will go a long way toward securing engagement and positive, constructive interaction. Blaming the client for any problems within the therapeutic relationship is contraindicated. It is the responsibility of the clinician, the professional, to build a therapeutic relationship. Our ethical standards insist on it; but more importantly, the outcome for our client depends on it.

Too often, clinical work gets off to a poor start because the assessment writer presents a very "diagnostic," problem-focused report, expressing an opinion from the professional evaluator "hat" as fact while disregarding or minimizing input from the client. The client's perspective of history and circumstances, and the full context around behaviors, are left out. A diagnosis based on brief interaction or testing without consideration of culture or current circumstances drives the recommendations. Many assessment writers are "medical model" rather than client centered and client-need driven. Client-centered and client-need-driven assessments will involve agreement and joint ownership of the report and the goals, which will assist the assigned therapist in engaging the client and working quickly to achieve desired outcomes.

Assessment as intervention is discussed in Chapter 5, where the story of Tom and his mother illustrates the impact an assessment writer can have on the eventual outcome.

The Client's Philosophy of Change Drives the Intervention

Our family and cultural upbringing, coupled with our life experiences, have cemented in us a belief of how change happens, as well as what needs to happen for significant change to occur. Clinical intervention is more effective when we can match the intervention to our client's belief of how real change occurs. A roadmap to a client's philosophy of change can be envisioned when we elicit client narratives around times when they have had a problem or challenge that has been resolved, perhaps similar to the presenting problem. In families, we need to be cautious because there can be cultural rules around change to which a therapist must adhere. For example, a parent's input or approval can be important before a child attempts certain behavioral changes, because in some family hierarchies there are values and codes of conduct requiring that change come through or be sanctioned by the head of the family.

Understanding what change looks like for our clients and how they see change happening enhances our alliance with them and increases the likelihood of success. It is critical that the client is the key to how the professional interacts. For example, if cheerleading and compliments have the opposite effect, then rather than cheerlead or compliment, thank your client for finishing an assignment. (For clients with reactive attachment issues, including some adopted children, praise can often backfire; but thanking them for a good effort is usually well accepted.) Every client is different, and "change processes" as well as "language" must be customized to fit the client.

There are Exceptions to Every Problem

Another concept connected to a client's philosophy of change that will help the change process to occur quickly involves "exceptions." Exceptions are about the times when the problem is not happening. There are exceptions to every problem, and clinicians need to help clients identify exceptions. If we accept that no problem is 24/7, we can ask the client to talk about times when the problem was not happening—what day, what hour, and what happened instead. The process with an individual client might go like this:

Client: I'm always depressed. My life sucks. It's horrible.
Therapist: So, what days last week did you feel a little better?
Client: I was depressed every day.
Therapist: Yikes! That must have been really difficult. It is a tribute to your strength that you are able to be here today. Let me ask: there must have been a day—or maybe part of a day—when things were a little bit better? Just a little better?
Client: Maybe Tuesday. Maybe Tuesday evening, when my daughter had her recital.
Therapist: Really. I want to hear all about the recital; but first, let me ask: what helped you to lift the depression, maybe just a little? What helped?
Client: Whenever I am with my kids, I feel better. I feel good. I miss them. This custody arrangement doesn't work. Every other weekend is an awful arrangement. I need more time with them.
Therapist: From our discussion last week during intake, it is clear that you are a great dad. You love your children—cherish them—and they are fortunate to have you in their life. Tell me, other than physically being around them, when does your depression lift? What helps?
Client: When I talk to them on the phone after work, that makes my evenings better. Really better, I guess. I need to know

they are okay. I worry about them, with the divorce and everything.

Therapist: Wow—as I said, you are a great dad. Having a father like you will give them a great foundation to grow. So, what needs to happen for you to be able to call them after work?

Client: I worry that I shouldn't call them too much. Maybe it will sadden them—remind them of the divorce. I guess I would have to know it's okay to check on them; that they are okay with me calling. I want what is best for them.

Therapist: I see. You want what is best for them. That makes sense. So that I can better understand, because I have never met your children, tell me about a time you called them and you knew it was a good thing to do, for them and for you. And then I want to hear about the recital!

The process with a couple might go like this:

Wife: I don't think he really cares. He's not considerate. He never thinks about me. We argue all the time. All I want is for him to care about me. It's like I don't matter to him.

Therapist: Tell me about a time when your husband was a little more considerate.

Wife: Well, hardly ever; but actually, he called me at work the other day to ask if I was okay.

Therapist: Oh—that's what you said you wanted, for him to be more sensitive to your feelings. [To husband] How did you know to do that?

Husband: Well, I knew she was worried about her performance evaluation, so I called her.

Therapist: You don't normally call her at work?

Husband: I usually don't think about it. I don't like to call. But I remembered that she said it would be a hard day for her, and that she didn't know how she would get through it. And I guess that was on my mind.

Therapist: So, you called because you thought she would need your support?

Husband: Yes; but if it was me, I would have wanted to be left alone. I don't think to call unless I am asked, or maybe if there is an emergency. We're different that way.

Therapist: I get it. You wouldn't think to call unless it was an emergency, or unless she told you that it would be important. One thing that I'm wondering is—how come it was on your mind this time?

Wife [interrupting]:	That was really nice of you. It was very important to me. I was thinking that it didn't matter to you; that you didn't think about what I was going through.
Therapist:	I hear that. And [your husband] was thinking about you that day. It was different. It was what you wanted him to do. You said that is really important to you! [To husband] So how come it was on your mind to call her yesterday?
Husband:	Well, I guess that I take words seriously—I mean, she told me that she needed support. I'm a sucker for following through with things I'm told are needed—like at work, or if something at home needs to be fixed. But I need to be asked directly, or I don't think about it. But once I am told something is wrong or important, it haunts me like it is my duty. I want to do the right thing, especially for my wife. She just expects it to be automatic; but it's not that I don't care. I can't read minds. I don't always get that it is so important; but if I'm told, I will call.
Wife:	Now I understand our arguments about you not being considerate. But I wish we wouldn't have to go through all this. I want you to call or be there when I need you.
Therapist [to the couple]:	What needs to happen next for you both to avoid going through this ordeal?

Sometimes we have to prompt an answer by telling the client that there must have been a time when the problem was not happening, or was less of a problem. After clarifying with the client details of the day or hours without the problem, it is important to give the client credit and reinforce the exceptions by processing with questions such as:

- "How did you do that?"
- "How did you know to do that?"
- "What helped?"
- "What was good about that?"
- "What needs to happen for more of that to happen?"

Complimenting and cheerleading help encourage the client to continue the effort. Tasks that create deliberate exceptions—in other words, exceptions to the problem that occur by conscious will or design as part of a task—can be effective in beginning a process of lasting change for clients.

It is surprising how often exceptions to the problem occur for our clients. Exceptions to every problem can be found or created to build solutions; and later, we will discuss methods for helping a client to create exceptions, as well as how to transition from problem talk to exceptions and solutions. The important thing to keep in mind is that when the exception is happening, the problem is not. The solution and problem cannot be happening at the same time. And it is not necessary to know the cause or the function of the client complaint in order to resolve it (O'Hanlon and Weiner-Davis 1989, pp. 38-39)—so feel free to take off that psychodynamic hat.

Clients often are so caught up in their problems that they do not notice when exceptions occur until we question them about it. As clinicians, we need to proceed ahead from what change will look like, and exceptions are a good indicator more times than not. The questions, "How did you do that?" and "What needs to happen for you to do more of that?" are excellent tools to move forward with process questions leading to the change the client wants. Transitioning from problem talk to exceptions to solution talk brings a cascade of hope and behavioral change for clients; but we must consciously use the client's exact words, the client's definition of the problem, and the client's experiences with the problem. The client's experiences, characterizations, and exact words need to be at the core of our intervention.

Change is Happening All the Time

Change is happening all the time. We are a little different every day, affected by circumstances and experiences, thoughts and behaviors, and the environment around us. Even a 50-minute visit to our therapist's office, a serious meeting with our boss, or a night out with a friend will have an impact on us—positive or negative. One of the significant concepts to remember is that small change can lead to larger change. A cornerstone in client-centered and solution therapies is that charting and then noticing incremental change as it occurs will empower clients to move in a direction to complete goals. It begins with a clear, behavioral goal that has come from what the client really wants—in other words, the client's agenda. Best practice in goal setting includes defining goals with small increments or steps that may take up to three weeks to complete. When the completion of each increment is in the client's control and the client has the resources needed, success is likely.

To be helpful as a catalyst for change, it is incumbent for therapists to learn incremental change thinking and processing. Later, through client narratives, we will explore several solid practice ideas to identify small changes and build on them, including scaling techniques that empower clients to recognize and pursue small (incremental) changes. For now, it is important to keep in mind that small changes occur frequently, and we often miss them if we do not have a strategy to recognize them.

One idea to help clients identify change that has already happened involves tasks or homework. Let's say that we elicit and then assign a task for a client to complete, and the client reports that they did not do it. Rather than leave it at that, we could inquire, "What part of the task did you do?" or "What did you do instead?" Thus, we have an opportunity to learn about something that was "different" and involved change, rather than blaming the client for not following through with our task. In later chapters, through stories that feature real client examples, we will detail ideas and strategies for promoting and recognizing meaningful change.

Cooperation is Inevitable

In client-centered and client-need-driven work, resistance is not a useful concept. We know that when we work from a client's agenda, and elicit rather than tell clients what to do, clients will become customers of change. In fact, clients are showing us how change takes place if we position ourselves to hear them. Blaming a client for our lack of skill is defeatist and counterproductive; but unfortunately, it happens among clinicians. One interesting way of looking at a client's apprehension comes from motivational interviewing. In motivational interviewing, resistance is not a central concept because ambivalence is looked at as a natural part of the change process. A lack of understanding or insensitivity by a counselor or therapist can easily sabotage the change process. I would advocate for clinicians to ask themselves, "What might I be missing?"

We need to accept that not all clients will be customers over therapy or the reasons for referral; and in fact, clients can be visitors or complainants over any issue or over therapy in general. Trying to work with a visitor or complainant as if they are a customer will rupture the therapeutic alliance and can cause harm. The good news is that there are practical, best practice ideas to work with clients who might be visitors or complainants; we will address them in another chapter. For now, let's define the three "positions" clients can take in general toward therapy, or toward any particular issue in therapy (Berg 1989).

Visitors do not think they have a problem. They do not know why they are there or what the value of the meeting might be. They seem indifferent; it's not their idea to receive services. A visitor will not do observational or behavioral change tasks, set authentic goals, or accept that participating in therapy will be worthwhile. The fact that they showed up matters and deserves a compliment. It is important that we use early session strategies with visitors to motivate them to come back for another meeting. This will be discussed in later chapters.

Complainants have a problem that cannot be solved. They complain about circumstances or other people. It is somebody else's fault. They are good at describing what is wrong but are challenged to find what makes it better. Complainants are great observers and will do observational tasks but not behavioral tasks. Working with complainants by listening, validating their concerns, acknowledging their strengths, identifying exceptions and how change will look, and learning about their agenda(s) will build a solid therapeutic foundation.

Customers have a problem they are trying to solve and are willing to work to change something. Working from their agenda(s) will keep them engaged as customers. Customers will do both observational and behavioral change tasks. We can usually help to move clients into a customer position through client-centered and client-need-driven solution work that prioritizes their agenda and builds a therapeutic atmosphere and collaborative relationship.

Appendix C features a summary of the positions a client can take toward therapy in general or issues in therapy.

Keep in mind that a client's initial receptiveness is not necessarily indicative of outcome. A client can be a visitor in relation to one issue, a complainant in relation to a second issue, and a customer in relation to a third issue. All clients will be customers in relation to their real agenda. When we can capture the moment and give a client hope and confidence, the client will be motivated to engage in therapy. In later chapters, we will discuss intervention strategies to build client hope and confidence.

Our services should be tailored to fit the client's position, so it is important to notice the client's position throughout the intervention. Asking clients to set goals, identify increments of change, or complete tasks must be in consideration of their position. We need to stop blaming clients for our lack of skills and find a way to better cooperate with them around their position. When we err, make assumptions, and get ahead of the client, we need to consider the results as feedback for us, and do something different.

In most cases, it will require skilled process work over several meetings for therapists and clients to work into solutions and resolution. There are situations, however, where clients can achieve their goals through a single task. Listening carefully to elicit the client's agenda, philosophy of change, and willingness to do what they say they want can open the door to a single session breakthrough. It also helps when clients are already partially doing their solution, even if they do not notice it. In general, anytime we listen to what a client really wants and help them to notice that they are already doing some of it or introduce a task that will accomplish what they want, the outcome will almost certainly be successful for them. Fifteen-year-old Vicki and her mother are prime examples of how this can work.

Teenage Vicki and Complainant Mom

A mother and her 15-year-old daughter were referred to me by a therapist who said that she was exhausted by the mother's complaining and the adolescent's arguing. The therapist's "file" indicated that she had seen mom and daughter together for six sessions after meeting with mom alone for an initial assessment. At the time of referral, the family's insurance company allowed me one intake session and asked that I justify the need for additional sessions. Progress notes in the referral packet indicated that the referring therapist had worked with mom and Vicki on communication and trust issues, conceptualizing the presenting problem as "adolescence" and "inconsistent parenting." Her prognosis for them was "grim," even though both mom and Vicki insisted on continuing therapy. My impression was that there was hope because both clients wanted to continue to work toward resolution.

I proposed to the insurance company that I would require four sessions to address unresolved issues around cooperation and solution building, and up to two additional follow-up appointments 90 days after the fourth session to confirm and consolidate continued progress. Part of my justification was that "adolescence was not something I could cure," and "from the notes I had received, it looked as if mom's parenting was very consistent, just not effective." I proposed that I would need to understand mom's "complaining" and would set goals that would address her complaints, reduce arguing, and enhance cooperation between mom and Vicki. Managed care authorized only three sessions plus the two follow-up sessions I requested.

When I met with mom and Vicki for our first appointment, it felt as if I was meeting with a more complicated family than the referring therapist had described. I listened carefully as Mom described her overwhelm as a single parent, working full-time, and burdened with fear for Vicki's wellbeing. She emphasized concerns regarding her daughter's maturation and the importance of life lessons to help Vicki become a responsible adult. Mom's indicator of her success or failure as a parent, as well as for Vicki's maturation, was the condition of the house—primarily that chores would be completed, the house would be clean, and she and Vicki would cooperate and jointly make an effort to keep up with their responsibilities. It was clear that mom's agenda was for the chores to be completed jointly, and the house to be orderly and clean. She did not believe that Vicki was cooperating with the important household chores. Mom presented as a complainant.

Vicki disagreed with mom's characterization of her level of cooperation and effort. Vicki insisted that she helped a lot and did more than her share, but it was never enough, because mom "never noticed what and how much" she had done. Vicki saw the problem as mom "not noticing"; and her agenda was for mom to notice her effort and what she did around the house every day. Vicki said that she would do anything to make that happen. Vicki presented as a customer in relation to mom noticing her efforts; and Vicki's solution was for mom to come home from work and acknowledge the chores that Vicki had completed. Her belief was that once mom acknowledged her effort and the work she had completed, mom would "calm down and maybe have a life."

We transitioned from problem talk to a process that elicited exceptions, although the exceptions were limited and conditional:

Mom: Sure, Vicki, when your friends are coming over you clean your room; but that doesn't count as cooperation. And that's just your room. I just need to see that you can make more of an effort.

Vicki: Mom, that is just not true. I clean every day. I want to keep the house clean. You just don't notice. Except maybe when I point it out to you. If even one time you just noticed the effort I made to help, I might feel appreciated. That's all I want.

Exception questions and fast-forward questions were answered, but met with some skepticism. The tune was akin to, "Show me; put up or shut up." This issue caused a great deal of stress and hurt between them. They both wanted resolution and to appreciate one another; but they were tired of the struggles. I could see that they were becoming impatient with each other and with answering my questions.

Both mom and Vicki had been customers in relation to therapy in general, yet they were frustrated over being stuck in a behavioral sequence of:

Vicki does chores to keep up the house /Mom comes home and says that she needs more help and Vicki hasn't been helping around the house / Vicki tells mom that she is being not appreciated and begins to tell mom what she has done /Mom cuts her off and complains to Vicki that there is so much to do and she needs help /Vicki insists that she does a lot and wants the same thing that mom wants /Mom disagrees and talks about her overwhelm and concern for Vicki's future as a responsible adult / Vicki tells mom that she's doing fine and wants things to work out well / Mom says that she is afraid that neither of them are in a good place and complains about a lack of cooperation and commitment.

Clearly, with a limited number of sessions and a lack of progress in therapy previously, they needed to address and find resolution for this issue sooner rather than later. Solution-focused question sequences are powerful and usually will take clients to resolution, but it was time to do something different. Solution work is very much about helping the client to accomplish what they want. I could see the opportunity to resolve this issue quickly because they told me exactly what they wanted. As a complainant in relation to the issue that was driving her agenda, I knew that mom might be receptive to complete observational tasks. Vicki, on the other hand, was a customer in relation to the issues behind her agenda and thus could be willing to do both observational and behavioral tasks. Their answer to my question, "What needs to happen for you to say that this problem has been resolved?" gave me an idea for a task; but there was still tension between Vicki and mom that needed to be addressed.

Tasks requiring participation of two or more clients are better received when there is an atmosphere of agreement and cooperation between the parties. Clearly, a little cooperation would lighten the mood and perhaps build hope. Adding some "intrigue" can be helpful and can even create a playful mood. To initiate this process and put them on the same page, I began with:

> It's a positive sign that each of you have clearly expressed agreement about what you want and what needs to happen to resolve your concerns. You've given me an idea for a task that would help, but I'm sort of reluctant to bring it up, this being only the first session.

They looked at me with inquisitive stares, and mom said, "What are you saying?" Then Vicki chimed in: "Let's hear it—why not?" I paused a moment before clarifying things:

> I want a commitment from you that you will take this seriously, and that you are sincerely invested in solving the problem that brought you here. I'd feel better telling you the task after knowing that I had a commitment.

Each of them timidly agreed at first; and after some reassurance to mom that it wasn't "kinky," they each said they would at least try it. Mom added, "Guaranteed"; and Vicki said, "I swear, I promise." So, I assigned them their task as follows:

> Vicki, you are saying that you do more than your share around the house. Here's a chance to prove it. I want you to secretly pick two days before our next appointment to be absolutely perfect and do more than

your share—much more. But don't tell your mom. If she says something like, "It's today, isn't it?", you have to lie to her and deny it. Keep
a list of everything you do on each of the two days and don't let your
mom see it. Keep it hidden and bring the list into the office for our next
appointment. You've been saying that you do a lot, so I want to hear
exactly what you did that your mom would like.

And mom, you have said that you would notice the things that Vicki
does to help if she really helped; so I want you to keep a list of all the
helpful things she does every day around the house between now and our
next appointment. From your list, figure out and write down which two
days she was trying to be perfect. I will ask you at our next appointment
to identify the two days, and then to read out loud everything she did to
be perfect, and we'll compare it to her list. This is your chance to show
her that you do notice. Keep your list secret and hidden from her.

Both mom and Vicki again agreed to complete their parts of the task—in
fact, quite enthusiastically. After the task was assigned, I asked them to
confirm: "On a willingness scale of 0-10, how willing are each of you to
complete the task?" Both confirmed a 10. "On a confidence scale, how
confident are each of you that both will complete the task?" Again, both
indicated a 10. The reason for these scales is to check if there is a potential
obstacle to completing the task—for example, mom may have business
appointments every evening next week, or Vicki may be focused on final
exams. If willingness or confidence is scaled as less than a 9, I ask clients
how the task can be modified to make it a 9 or 10.

Mom and Vicki returned for their next appointment nine days later and
were noticeably excited when they took their seats. I began the session
with the general question, "What's better?" Mom held up a several-page
list of the chores Vicki had completed that she had noticed and said,
"It was Tuesday and Wednesday, wasn't it?" Vicki held up her list and
blurted out, "No, mom—Tuesday and Thursday." I replied, "Wow, that's
great! I want to hear, mom, what you noticed on Tuesday and compare
it with Vicki's list; but first, I am really interested in what you noticed
Vicki did to help on Wednesday—a day she wasn't just doing chores for
the task."

They both enthusiastically shared their lists, and it was clear that the
interactions between them were much improved. Mom also was able to
recall the chores Vicki had claimed on Thursday even though she had
not initially listed them as occurring on one of the "be perfect" days.
Compliments were shared and they sounded closer, upbeat, and confident
that there was resolution. The tension in the office had lifted and mom
and Vicki looked into each other's eyes with a clear sense of fondness and
appreciation.

The dynamics of this task probably create an incentive to do more and notice more, which is exactly what Vicki and her mom said they wanted. Vicki's agenda was for mom to notice and acknowledge when she helped around the house. Through completion of the task, mom demonstrated that she could notice and appreciate what Vicki had done to help around the house. Mom's agenda was for the chores to be completed jointly, and the house to be orderly and clean. Vicki showed through the task that she could complete the chores that mom regarded as important. They cooperated and both of their agendas were met. Vicki saw that she could trust mom to notice. They were both customers in relation to therapy and the issues we were addressing.

We scheduled another meeting to process some of mom's concerns about the future of teenagers in general and her daughter specifically, and then followed up with a session several months later. The conflicts over responsibility and cooperation had subsided. Both Vicki and mom indicated that things were resolved between them. It was clear that at least some of mom's fears about her daughter were assuaged.

For some problem-focused therapists, instead of discharge, mom might have been diagnosed with anxiety, and additional sessions would be scheduled for her to work on fears about her daughter's future and whatever else came out of those discussions. Vague, somewhat non-specific issues are what can keep clients in therapy for months or even years. My plan was to offer them a follow-up session anytime in the future if there was something that concerned either of them. When I do not hear back from clients, I follow up with a phone contact at 90 days to confirm things are still on track. In this case, mom and Vicki were continuing to cooperate and were getting along fine. Their outlook and mood over cooperation and chores had profoundly improved merely from the experience of completing the task. Just doing the solution can have lasting effects.

When we trust our clients as the experts, consider their agenda and positions toward issues and generally toward therapy, and elicit their solutions to the problem, successful intervention does not have to be complicated. Through tasks that feature what they want to see happen, clients can be incentivized to participate and practice their solutions. We can ask about and process exceptions to the problem or create "deliberate exceptions" through tasks. Too often, therapists are the resistant ones, insisting that clients accept and pursue certain prescribed goals or benchmarks. There are several books or articles that cite successes with referrals of another therapist's "difficult" or "impossible clients." Clinicians who insist on being the expert on the client's life or who predict the likelihood of success based on the client's history, initial receptiveness, or diagnosis are creating dynamics that can sabotage cooperation and outcomes. We discuss this further in Chapter 4.

References

Berg, I. K. (1989). Of visitors, complainants, and customers: Is there really such a thing as Resistance? *Family Therapy Networker*, *13* (1).

O'Hanlon, W. and Weiner-Davis, M. (2003). *In Search of Solutions*. New York: Norton.

Rogers, C. (1961). *On Becoming a Person*. New York: Houghton Mifflin Company.

4 Expectancy and Hope
Treatment Considerations and Outcomes

Very early in my career, I accepted a temporary grant position as a counselor for "Children in Need of Supervision" (CHINS), a status assigned to adolescents who were non-violent juvenile offenders with a mental health diagnosis. Most of the adolescents had been removed from their parents' home and were living in "specialized care foster homes," under the dual supervision of Juvenile Probation and Child Welfare. My previous clinical experience outside of internships had involved crisis counseling with substance-using adolescents and their families.

On paper, I may have met the minimum qualifications to provide counseling for a caseload of CHINS adolescents and families with multiple issues; but in actuality, I was lacking some of the sophistication that would have been helpful when addressing families with overwhelming behavioral, socioeconomic, and legal challenges. The counseling was complex: intervene with the adolescent's family to encourage court-mandated steps toward reunification; address the adolescent's behavior and mental health issues; and work closely with the Juvenile Court and Child Welfare. The good news from those experiences is that I learned an unexpected yet valuable lesson, which would make me a more effective therapist, mental health supervisor, and clinical manager in the future.

On my first day at work, Peggy, my new supervisor, convened a meeting for me to meet my coworkers and receive a job orientation. We sat in a circle, and following a brief introduction, each of the experienced clinicians provided me with an overview of the job from their perspective. They detailed "dos and don'ts"; and they shared insights regarding the court, foster care agency, juvenile justice, and mental health programming, as well as procedural "beartraps" to avoid. Staff emphasized that despite having to service clients with complex issues who were receiving scrutiny from multiple agencies, the program "saved a lot of kids." There was a great deal of energy and pride among the staff. At the end of the orientation, my new supervisor said, "So that Saul can get off to a running start, I need each of you give him four or five of your case files and let me know

DOI: 10.4324/9781003397380-4

who they are." No doubt you can imagine the histories and dynamics of the cases I received! When I left the program a couple of years later, one of my coworkers recalled my first day and admitted that those cases were "the clients from hell."

My employer, receiving public monies as part of the state welfare system, maintained careful outcome and expense records. There were three sections that monitored and tracked services and expenses: Eligibility, Welfare, and Child Welfare. Clients were tracked every quarter and at year-end. Interestingly, my results with those "impossible clients" were no different than the results for the clients that my coworkers had chosen to keep for themselves. Why? From the start, I accepted the youth and families as MY CLIENTS! They were going to do well because I was going to help them. I believed in them. I had hope for them and, perhaps more importantly, they had attained hope for themselves with the assignment of a new counselor. I expected success, and they could see and hear confidence and enthusiasm in my presentation. We were going to do great things together! There is power in what we believe and what we expect.

Thus, I was fortunate early in my career to recognize the power in expectancy—not only the therapist's expectancy, but also the client's expectancy about the therapist and the potential outcome. Several years later, I came across a reference that discussed the profound impact of expectancy on a client's hope for a good outcome (O'Hanlon and Weiner-Davis 1989, pp. 33-34). I must conclude that more important than what the therapist actually believes about the probable outcome for the client is the client's belief about what the therapist believes. As I have refined my thinking and reflected on my experiences, my conclusion is that expectancy is a primary factor in building a solid foundation for hope. Hope from a client's perspective and hope from a therapist's perspective can together be essential for a good outcome. It is incumbent on the therapist to find a way to communicate an optimistic and hopeful outlook to the client, as well as to honestly maintain genuine hope for the client.

What a client believes the therapist believes is probably less stable than any of the other factors that interplay with hope and expectancy. Both positive expectancy and hope can be challenged by a client setback. A therapist's attitude and how a client setback is processed, as well as the wording of questions after a setback, are critical factors that will influence the ultimate outcome. In the last section of this chapter, we discuss proven strategies for therapists to implement following a client setback.

Later in my career, as a supervisor or clinical manager, when an intern or clinician would complain about a client or otherwise lose hope, I would consider reassigning that client. My preferred strategy in those situations was to meet with both the existing clinician and a neutral clinician in order to brainstorm a way they could be genuine and facilitate hope. This would afford a teaching moment to work with the original intern or clinician around "what needs to happen in order to build and maintain hope with and for your clients." My goal was for "fresh eyes" to help restore the therapist-client relationship, and have it anchored in mutual hope and confidence. Only if that was not possible would I reassign the client-family to the new therapist.

Hope, willingness, and confidence are key elements of the therapeutic process. Ensuring that our clients maintain hopeful and confident attitudes and beliefs throughout therapy is one of the keys to success. Keeping a pulse on the client's outlook and willingness to work toward change, even when there are setbacks, can help us to remove potential roadblocks to success before they become entrenched. It is the therapist's responsibility to establish the therapeutic alliance and learn whatever it will take to empower the client.

Traditional Medical Model Psychiatry Can Work Against the Power of "Hope"

Medical model approaches in psychotherapy are quite different than client-centered, client-need-driven, strength-based approaches. In the medical model paradigm, the professional is the expert and identifies the problem, "prescribes" interventions, and designs solutions. The client is seen as responsible for the situation and is required to be compliant and follow the recommendations of the professional. Language and the "definition of the problem" are often based on the *Diagnostic and Statistical Manual of Mental Disorders*. Disagreement with the professional "expert" is called "resistance." Conversely, in a client-centered or client-need-driven approach, such as the social constructivist or "solution-focused" model, the relationship between the clinician and client is collaborative. The professional is not a diagnostician independent of the client, and notices the client's strengths and resources as opportunities, rather than focusing only on deficits and barriers.

There have been studies, books, and articles written about "impossible clients." Those studies usually look at clients who had been seeing "medical model" psychiatrists or psychologists and were diagnosed with at least one (what used to be referred to as Axis II) personality disorder in addition to a mental health disorder. The original practitioner would identify certain clients as "impossible," and then a client-centered therapist would work with those clients. As you can probably guess, those clients turned out to not be "impossible" under a different approach—one that began with an expectancy around success and focused on client strengths and solutions.

During my marriage and family therapy licensing internship, one of my assignments was to work for a few weeks in a hospital with an inpatient mental health wing. Every week a treatment team was facilitated by one of the psychiatrists. Usually present were a licensed clinical social worker, psych techs, psych nurses, and one or more psychologists. As the psychiatrist reviewed each name from a patient chart, he would comment and then ask those working with or monitoring the patient to add their feedback, prognosis, and recommendations. Occasionally, he would get to a patient chart and extend his arm up, with his index and middle finger pointing toward the ceiling in what looked like a "V." I noticed that none of the team members had offered intervention ideas and a prognosis in their summaries for those patients. After that first treatment team, I asked one of the psychologists what the "V" sign meant. "It's not a 'V' sign," I was told. "It means Axis II." The message was that there was no hope for a patient with a diagnosis of a personality disorder, so why bother?

I have heard similar stories from peers who did inpatient work in the 1960s through the early 2000s. In many settings, the diagnosis became a self-fulfilling prophecy. There are still clinicians who were trained in this way of thinking and continue to practice it. We know better from experience with clients over time. Looking at behaviors and engaging a client's strengths and resources to overcome issues and problems is far more effective than being driven by a diagnostic label. Skilled practitioners can help clients to impact the behaviors that, in combination, resulted in their diagnosis. It saddens me to think that there are clients who have been, and even today continue to be, neglected or pathologized because of negative expectancy from their treatment personnel.

Appendix D outlines the differences between the medical model and the constructivist model.

Our Downtown Offices Can Be Uncomfortable for Clients

There is another facet of expectancy that can have a profound effect on client outcomes. Clients who live in surroundings or have a family history that is dramatically different than their therapist's life experiences can feel vulnerable, and in fact can be subjected to stereotyping by community resources, agencies, or therapists. Some clients who come to our "downtown offices" from areas that are socioeconomically and culturally different, perhaps mandated to treatment with much to lose, can feel out of place—even on trial. We might inaccurately judge them because we see an "out-of-context" snapshot of their life, not the more accurate full-length movie.

Seeing disadvantaged, fragile, and vulnerable families in their homes could provide a very different picture and reveal strengths and opportunities for change that may not be apparent when they are outside their natural environment. It is for these reasons and others that "in-home" therapy can have advantages for better engagement and lasting outcomes. If in-home therapy is not possible, appointments at a community resource center in a client's neighborhood, perhaps with family or "fictive kin" participating, can be advantageous over a downtown or suburban therapist's office. "Fictive kin" are discussed in Chapter 6.

Conversely, clients might inaccurately judge and stereotype a therapist. They could find it hard to accept that we understand them, accept them, really like them, and can be helpful. They might picture our personal history as a life without adversity or struggles, and instead filled with advantages and privilege. We need to be careful about too much personal disclosure, especially in high-security settings. What I have learned from clients is that finding a way to break through even a small slice of a stereotype can open the door to earn trust as someone who might be helpful; and that being humble and compassionate goes a long way in therapy. It is important for therapists to figure out what is getting in the way of engagement and trust, and to take responsibility for finding an appropriate way to make things better.

When I worked at the Department of Prisons, I was assigned to provide psychotherapy services in both a men's and women's medium-security correctional center. There are stringent rules around self-disclosure and information sharing due to security and safety concerns. During our first three weeks of employment, we were required to complete mandatory training in the dangers of working in a secure, locked correctional facility. We learned that groups of inmates "study staff" and share information with the goal of obtaining leverage to manipulate favors. Anything inmates learn about your personal life can be exploited through a friend or relative of theirs in your community. It was surprising to see how frequently staff were compromised, losing their jobs and, in several cases, even their freedom. Nurses, psychologists, correctional officers, maintenance staff, and even a warden were compromised and arrested during the seven years I worked there.

In the 1980s and 1990s, there were two men's prisons and one women's prison in Carson City. A federal lawsuit brought against Nevada by inmate Alan Taylor resulted in the hiring of a significant number of medical and mental health personnel throughout the state prison system. Working in a prison provides a daily reminder of the stark contrast between our lives "on the outside" and the survival needs of the inmates. Joining with inmates yet attending to issues around trust and safety requires a somewhat different mindset and comfort level. In the hierarchy of the inmate world, we were regarded as potential tickets for drugs, escape, early release, or parole considerations. Your workday began with the clang of a steel door behind you and a reminder that entering the "yard" meant that if you were taken hostage, preventing escape was worth more than your life.

Clients May Have a Sanitized Image of Who We Are

Unsurprisingly, compared to the men, a higher number of women inmates were more willing to voluntarily seek therapy. There were some inmates who participated wholeheartedly in therapy from the beginning; they were often from middle-class backgrounds or in prison for "white-collar" crimes. Then there were a number of inmates who did not see clinicians as inhabitants of a planet with the same "thinking" as them. Unless they felt understood and were addressed in a non-threatening way, their expectancy bias worked against therapeutic process. In other words, if a client expects to be negatively judged, misunderstood, even ridiculed, they adopt an attitude of:

> Because you cannot possibly understand or have compassion for me, I am not going to interact with you. You have to prove to me that you are not that person I imagine you are—even though you look like the picture of entitlement, prejudice, and judgment.

Obviously, there are serious challenges to joining and engaging when a client stereotypes a clinician as having experienced a sanitized, privileged life filled with advantages and opportunities.

One of the women inmates who seemed to be aloof toward the therapeutic process would visit and chat casually and freely with me when my office door was open. Vivian, aka "Viper," told me about her cynical view of the world, her children, and her love of ice cream: "Vanilla or chocolate; I know it's strange, but equally good to me." She shared her belief that "life is unfair if you don't have money." One day she said that she thought I was a good guy, but I could never understand and help her—or, for that matter, anyone she knew. Her reasoning was that I lived in a privileged dimension and could not understand a life different than my own. I asked her to describe minute to minute what she thought I would see and do when I left the prison that evening. She replied:

> You will go through the office and security gate; probably chat a little, maybe flirt with the female officers on your way out; get into your Mercedes; put in a tape of classical music, keep the windows closed and turn up the music; drive on the freeway—no, speed to your house in the mountains; get home to your wife and kids; pour a glass of fine wine …

After hearing that description, I understood her expectation that I could never relate to anything in her life. Her picture of my person, my likes, and my life was not accurate. In fact, I found it disturbing because I would never have imagined that anyone could picture me that way. But I understood that perception matters, and it was up to me to find a way to be genuine and honest, show positive regard, and constructively connect with her and her peers if I was to interest them in therapy. For Viper to have hope and the expectation of success should she ever become a client, she had to have faith in me; and the idea that I was a Mercedes owner and classical music "nerd" who lived in the mountains and did not have a human bone in my body was prohibitive to her. (And for the record, there was no Mercedes—I drove a Toyota; and I have never been a classical music fan.)

There was one way, perhaps, to alter at least part of my "image" that would be honest, genuine, and not create security issues or undesirable side effects. I was a fan of classic rock and contemporary rock and roll music. In community office settings, I listened to music while writing reports, clinical notes, or completing insurance forms. So, I brought in a "boombox" with some tapes or CDs of the Rolling Stones, the Beatles, and current hits of the 1980s, and played them in my office while doing paperwork. It worked. My client caseload increased considerably, and inmates were more open with personal disclosure. Viper eventually became a client and participated in therapy, making significant gains, earning parole, and eventually, I was told, living some of the changes she aspired to achieve.

When I reflected on this experience, I realized Viper was right. I could never have a deep understanding of her history and feelings—or the context of her experiences in her family. What I learned, however, is that living her experiences firsthand or not had nothing to do with whether I could be helpful or effective. The client is in the driver's seat. When Viper was able to risk disclosure, sharing her "definition of the problem" and responding to my questions about her "philosophy of change," "exceptions," and history of problem solving, therapy worked for her. Viper's testimonials brought dozens of inmates into therapy with me over the next few years.

Later in my career, I was able to reflect on this experience when supervising interns without children of their own were working with families. My interns shared their discomfort when clients asked them if they too had children. I promoted the idea of responding conceptually with:

> If you will teach me about your experience as a parent, and help me to understand what you want, maybe I can help you figure out what to do—but I understand that you are the expert on your family, so you need to teach me first about you and your children. I would never pretend to know better than you about you and your children.

Expectancy and the image or stereotype that clients have about their therapist are related. A client's hope, willingness, and confidence are at least partially based on a belief in the therapist and the therapist's ability to understand, accept, and be invested in the betterment of the client. When a client believes that a therapist could not understand, or is negatively judging the client, or does not think the client is worthy or capable, the client's expectation will work against a positive outcome. Remember, more important than what the therapist actually believes about the probable outcome for the client is the client's belief about what the therapist believes.

Create an Expectation of Success After a Setback

There are various schools of thought that normalize setbacks as "two steps forward, one step back." Certainly, as a reframe, that way of thinking can be productive and help a client to keep a focus on gains while perhaps avoiding self-condemnation over the setback. There is an additional way for a therapist to view a setback that I have found helpful in thinking about the future direction of therapy. In combination with the concept of setback as a temporary "one step back" challenge, I like to think of whatever occurred as "feedback, not failure." Learning from the experience, we can think about what else the client needed or would need to avoid a reoccurrence and stay on track.

One of the tenets of solution work is that clients define the problem, set their own goals, identify exceptions, and live their solutions. My first question when there is a client setback relates to whether the problem, goal, and solution belong to the client, or whether they were in some way inadvertently coerced by me or another person. If the client does not own the definition of the problem, goal, and solution, the setback could be because the change was about pleasing someone else or doing what they were told—in other words, "compliance" or "first-order change." It is also possible that other circumstances may have complicated the client's life and choices. Either way, I can attempt to reprocess the issues with the client in a non-shaming manner while communicating that the client is ultimately responsible for their choices.

Setbacks can function as both teaching moments and learning opportunities for therapists. There is a well-known excuse in golf after a golfer has putted a ball ten or more feet past the hole: "I fell in love with the line." It means that the golfer was so focused on the line they had envisioned for the putt to go into the hole that they forgot to consider the speed of the putt before stroking the ball. Likewise, therapists sometimes fall in love with their solution idea or a task, and do not consider other factors, including client willingness, confidence, resources, and comfort or compatibility. The result can be the therapist repeating a failed intervention or task again and again, despite the client not following through. The best feedback for a therapist is what a client actually does, not the "brilliance" of the intervention or task. Therapists need to be careful not to "fall in love" with their methodology, intervention strategy, or task, and miss the target.

Assessment Writers Highly Influence Expectancy

Whether it is an established client or a new client who has experienced the setback, it can be helpful to complete a short supplemental assessment and establish or perhaps reset some priorities and goals. The concept of a "fresh start" or "regrouping" might mark a hopeful beginning for a distressed client. For new clients, a history and cultural assessment is indicated. For existing clients, therapists can benefit from self-inquiry to reflect on and understand the following:

- "Was it their goal or mine that didn't work; or was it maybe someone else's plan?"
- "Who determined what the solution would look like?"
- "Did the client have all the resources needed?"
- "What is the client's hierarchy of needs?"
- "Are there other issues/limitations?"

Appendix E sets out process questions to use following a setback (Berg, I.K. and Miller 1992, pp.140-143).

In Chapter 5, the story of Johnny illustrates how to help create a hopeful beginning and initiate the solution process for a client who relapses, "hits bottom," and loses everything. In Johnny's intervention—as in Sarah's, outlined below—we can challenge a client's disparaging beliefs about themselves, the relapse, and the meaning of the relapse. Building hope and a positive expectancy bias for the client is critical. Many clients will initially look at their therapist as a critical parent and feel shame, even expecting condemnation; so it is imperative to help the client believe that the therapist is accepting and anticipates a good result. Therapists need to possess the maturity and skill to avoid judgment, be level, and take a position of advocacy with the client.

"I'm No Better than My Mother"

Sarah, a 24-year-old single mother, relapsed after 297 days of sobriety. During the 23 days of relapse, she lost her job and was unable to pay her current month's rent. She took her six-year-old daughter to her sister's house and entered a community residential rehabilitation treatment program for help. Sarah explained that she was afraid Child Welfare would take her daughter, Kati, so she made sure that Kati would be safe. Sarah's sister was self-supporting and never used substances, and according to Sarah, "has her life together."

We met with Sarah at the beginning of her second week in the program. The facility is a 28-day inpatient substance use disorder (SUD) treatment program. Sarah told us that previously, while in treatment there, the program had helped her to stay clean and sober for 297 days. During almost ten months of sobriety, she had worked and supported herself and her daughter. What was different this time was that Sarah had no hope and said that she always seemed to mess things up when life started to improve. She was feeling remorse and failure, believing that she was not worthy of having her daughter back because of the relapse.

Notably, Sarah talked about how her mother loved drugs more than she loved her and her sister, neglected them both when they were children, and had no desire to stop using. Sarah confided in us that she was bitter about how she had lost her childhood because she had to take care of her mother and sister. Sobbing, Sarah sheepishly said: "I'm no better than my mother. I've ruined my life and my daughter's future."

Clearly, substance abuse treatment alone would not be sufficient. Sarah shared that she was haunted by unresolved issues from childhood and feared that she was just like her mother. We knew that it would be critical to help her process the many ways in which she was different than her mother without demonizing her mother. Staff who worked with Sarah acknowledged her strengths as a parent to her daughter. It became pronounced, as she proceeded in treatment, that she was literally grieving—and had been for years—over parentification and the loss of her childhood.

Sarah's mother was a single parent who went to work and made an adequate income, but began to drink immediately after returning home from work. Sarah recalled writing rent checks for her mom when she was ten years old; walking to the grocery store four blocks from home to shop; and cooking, cleaning, and putting her sister to bed. Sarah's mother was a community liasion to the Police Department, and the neighborhood covered for her. No one was willing to call the authorities. Local merchants got to know Sarah and their family's situation, and would even allow her to buy cigarettes for her mother or cash her mother's checks without question.

Listening to Sarah and asking assessment questions, we were able to write down her issues as she expressed them to us. The following is a summary of what she told us:

- Addicted to substances;
- Lost hope;

- Feeling defeated;
- No confidence;
- Don't feel worthy of having a daughter;
- Afraid I am like my mother;
- History of periods of sobriety, followed by relapse;
- Anger over losing my childhood;
- Children deserve better than a mother who uses;
- Let everyone down;
- Proved again that I'm not worthy.

We respected Sarah's words as her core issues and concerns by writing them down exactly as she had stated them. At a later date—after discussion, clarification, reframing, exception questions, and some processing—we would support her in transitioning to goals. But for now, she needed to know that we had heard each item on the list, and understood her concerns. All concerns needed to be acknowledged, and some needed to be interpreted delicately. For example, "Proved again that I'm not worthy" would be processed on the spot as "fear that I am *no longer* worthy," after having her confirm—perhaps through a "soft" exception question—that she had felt worthy in the past. A skilled assessment professional would open the door to reframe "fear that I am no longer worthy" as "I am worthy and this is a setback," in order to create hope and additional possibilities for self-forgiveness, corrective actions, and healing. The caution here is not to step outside of the client's beliefs or reality too soon. My preference is to demonstrate an understanding of the client's concerns and sprinkle lots of hope and sincere compliments as you move forward.

During the assessment, we discussed Sarah's social and family history, cultural history, and substance use history, and elicited some of her strengths. It was important for her to partner with us and identify, then acknowledge strengths. Later, we discussed with her how those strengths would help her to heal and complete her goals. As Sarah continued in therapy, we assisted her in adding to the list of strengths. Reminding Sarah of her strengths and resources was a cornerstone to maintaining hope and confidence. Even the fact that she had remained in the program for two weeks at that time was significant. Assessment writers can err by focusing more on the problems than on strengths and the beginnings of change already in process. We did not make that error.

Strengths:

- Sober for 297 days prior to relapse.
- Entered treatment voluntarily. ("How did you decide to go to treatment?")

- Willing to work on issues.
- Complying with treatment.
- Job skills.
- Proven ability to be self-sufficient/hold job, meet expenses.
- Took daughter to sister's house voluntarily (protecting child).
- Loves her daughter.
- Two solid weeks in program (and counting).
- Program worked before for almost a year after discharge.
- Was there for her sister as child and is now making sure daughter is safe.
- Great caregiver/took care of mom and sister.
- Sister owes her good outcome to the strong guidance and care Sarah gave to her.
- Feels remorse.
- Well spoken.
- Knows how she wants things to be for herself and her daughter.
- Is meeting with you (you can say to a client, "You are here meeting with me").
- Is committed to treatment and staying sober.
- Already has shown that she is different than her mother.

First and foremost, we were there to demonstrate understanding, with clear communication that "we get it" after listening to "problem talk." Validation is a critical element as we hear our client's experiences. When she was ready, we were able to transition Sarah from problem talk to strengths and exception talk. Then we set goals and explored solutions with her through questioning and eliciting. It can be helpful to measure hope and confidence with questions, scaling, or other means. It was also helpful to communicate through words and actions that there was an expectation of success for Sarah as a parent and responsible, sober adult. Questions such as the following helped form the basis for compliments:

- "How did you stay sober for so long?"
- "How did you decide to do that?"
- "What do you know now that you didn't know before?"
- "When you are sober and in your own home for several months, what will be different?"

Setbacks can be opportunities to identify strengths, build hope, and establish or strengthen motivation for success. Clients will often feel vulnerable, discouraged, or hopeless after a setback. It is the therapist's mission to turn things around in a constructive, hopeful direction, and communicate a positive outlook. It is usually not productive to judge a client and initiate extensive discussions into patterns of failure. Rather, it is an opportunity to look at strengths and complete process work through difference questions, transition questions, and fast-forward questions about how recovery and healing will look. Crisis is often the best opportunity for intervention and change! (We discuss this further in Chapter 5.)

Sarah stabilized, acquired hope, developed an aftercare plan, and was discharged from the SUD treatment facility. She moved in with her sister temporarily and secured employment so that she could pay her share of the bills. Her aftercare plan included outpatient therapy, and Sarah attended sessions with me twice a month for almost six months, working on issues related to her history including childhood trauma, lack of confidence, addiction, and parenting concerns.

We learned that when Sarah was 17 years old, her mother was arrested for selling dangerous drugs. Sarah and her sister were placed with her deceased father's sister's family. Sarah left her aunt's home and moved in with a young man whom she had met at a fast-food restaurant where she was working. When Sarah became pregnant, he told her that he would be a father to Kati; but he never followed through with his promise. Sarah had mixed feelings about contacting him after so many years but said she would discuss it with Kati if she brought it up. It was clear that Sarah would be protective of Kati and try to act in her best interests.

Although Sarah came across as open and invested in therapy, and made progress, it always felt as if there were underlying hurts that were choking her emotionally. Then one day she decided to reveal the secret that had been shaming her. When she was ten years old, one of her mother's boyfriends raped her. Two other boyfriends also had sexual intercourse with her until she was 16. For six years she had protected her sister and kept the men away from her, sometimes through cooperating with or even initiating seduction. Sarah also told me that more than once she found it necessary to threaten one of the men with physical harm and disclosure if he touched her sister.

We reported the sexual abuse to the authorities and then I talked with Sarah about some options. A colleague of mine specialized in therapy with women who had endured sexual trauma as children, and Sarah eventually completed therapy with her. Sarah did well for herself, maintaining sobriety and working as a receptionist and an administrative assistant, eventually receiving a promotion to office manager. Years later, her daughter Kati completed college, excelling in graduate school, and began her career teaching at a community college and working in a counseling center. When Kati was hired, Sarah called me and said, "I have a great kid. I can't thank you enough for believing in us." (I found myself crying on and off over several days after receiving that call.)

It is our professional and ethical responsibility to keep a pulse on our client's expectations of themselves and their therapist, building trust and hope. Cheerleading, praise, and even a "Wow, you did it!" can be healthy for the therapeutic alliance. Most clients keep secrets from us, and sometimes it does not matter; but in Sarah's case, it mattered greatly that she finally revealed her painful secret. All the compliments and strength talk created an atmosphere that eventually made it safe for her to disclose. Clearly, treatment strategies that cement hope and demonstrate a therapist's expectation of client success are important to achieving good outcomes.

References

Berg, I.K., and Miller. (1992). *Working with the Problem Drinker: A Solution Focused Approach*. New York: Norton.
O'Hanlon, W., and Weiner-Davis, M. (1989). *In Search of Solutions*. New York: Norton.

5   Building a Positive, Hopeful Start
You Are More Than Your Problems

In addition to being the best opportunity for intervention, crisis is often a time ripe for engaging a client in the therapeutic process to facilitate change. When we can capture the moment and transition from a client's hopelessness and desperation to an atmosphere of hope and confidence, clients will be motivated to experiment with, if not engage in, therapy. Even when the situation and issues are such that the client is not ready to hear or benefit from exceptions and solutions, there are opportunities to set the stage for engaging, cheerleading, and motivating a client to become a customer in therapy.

Judgmental Interventions Can Be Counterproductive

When clients have suffered long-term recidivism, feelings of failure and hopelessness, and significant losses of people, property, and resources, and when they are faced with the possibility of severe consequences such as incarceration or loss of custody of their children, some clinicians choose interventions that are directive and confrontative. You might ask, "What better options do therapists have but to look to the circumstances as leverage and steer clients toward compliance as a means to help them?" After all, there are significant sanctions and losses associated with repeating offenses, violating court orders, or engaging in risky behaviors. Clients risk loss of freedom, loss of health, loss of family, loss of life, or outcomes that negatively affect others.

Based partially on that thinking, problem-focused and what I would call "moralistic" interventions that confront decisions and behaviors were developed many years ago. Those counseling models were used with adults and juvenile justice offenders for the purpose of confronting clients with the consequences of their choices. Unfortunately, those approaches tend to be shaming, judgmental, and insensitive to differences in culture, socioeconomics, and socialization; so there can be the potential for harm.

DOI: 10.4324/9781003397380-5

One downside of any therapy that "tells" or "confronts" is that compliance is not lasting, genuine change. Clients who leave therapy without making internal changes are prone to experience the same old counseling nightmare over and over:

> You are my fourth therapist in seven years ... I can't believe that I am having to do this again ... Things are worse than ever ... I lost my AA/NA chip and have to start all over ... I already tried that ... This time my life might really be over ... I'll do anything to stay out of prison but the judge has it in for me ... I will be different this time but no one will care ... Somehow I am going to get my kids back ... This time it wasn't my fault.

Good people, well-meaning and dedicated to helping clients, might be inadvertently recreating the same pattern for clients by using a "stale" approach. Too often clients experience the same interventions that do not work, or that only partially work, and find themselves either feeling like failures, hopeless and defeated, and/or thinking that therapy does not work. We need to be better than that. My approach includes ideas that evolved from Steve de Shazer's overarching tenant of solution-focused brief therapy (SFBT): "If it ain't broke don't fix it" (de Shazer & Dolan 2021 pp.1-2), and evolved into a widely accepted core philosophy of solution therapists:

- If it works, don't fix it. Do more of it.
- If it works a little, build on it.
- If it doesn't work, do something different (absurd, illogical, and unrelated to the problem is okay).
- Keep it simple.
- There is no failure—only feedback.
- Approach each visit as if it were the last (change is happening all the time, so engage the process).

Interpreted, the idea is to do "what works" or "build on what works a little bit" until you learn exactly what works for your client. It is better to "do something different" that breaks up a destructive pattern rather than trying the same thing over and over again. Sometimes a client can benefit from an idea or task that is not directly related to the problem. We need to keep it simple and uncomplicated instead of looking for some extravagant or complicated method. Whatever is "working" needs to be something that our client can replicate on their own, outside of therapy.

When our intervention is not working for the client, it is not "the client's fault." Rather than blame, we need to think of the result as simply feedback for us. If it did not work, we need to figure out with the client what will "work." And we need to approach each session as the last, acknowledging that it is our professional and ethical responsibility to leave our clients with whatever tools are necessary to help them complete their agenda and satisfy their goals. We can learn "what works" from an understanding of our client's family history, culture, agenda, definition of the problem, exceptions, and problem-solving history.

I listened carefully when clients who had "failed" in therapy two, three, or four times were referred to me, sometimes as a "last chance or else ..." Those clients described to me patterns of failed clinical interventions that included forced choices and behaviors. They were clear on what did *not* work in therapy:

- talking incessantly about the problem;
- referring to the court order as a reminder;
- a therapist's negative attitude and doomsday scenarios;
- treating group disclosures like Alcoholics Anonymous (AA) meetings (admit to your problems and powerlessness over your addiction);
- confrontations about history and mistakes;
- trying to extort change through "this way or else ..." choices;
- telling them what would be best for them, and what decisions to make;
- the therapist acting like they were better than the client and "judging" them; and
- blaming the client's parents and childhood caregivers.

Common to many descriptions of failed therapy was a mandated "agenda" based on satisfying the judge or referral source without sufficient consideration for the client's wants and needs. In those instances, the informed consent provisions, goals, and therapy were "referral source-need driven" rather than "client-need driven." Clients' stories revealed that they most often entered treatment as "visitors" in relation to therapy and found it challenging to become "customers." Their counselors or therapists were only marginally successful at completing engagement and getting client buy-in.

So how do you get a client with a pattern of losses in life and failures in therapy to look to the future with the optimism and energy needed to turn things around? We will look at strategies for joining and engaging; moving clients from being visitors or complainants to customers; using a client's expertise and history to create hope, willingness, and confidence; avoiding triangulation and splitting; and implementing proven client-need-driven interventions to diffuse the "power" of the problem.

"Our Group Is for Solution Building and Understanding"

For several years, in addition to my private practice, I had a contract with a community addiction and behavioral health treatment facility to provide group therapy services for dual diagnosis clients—those with co-occurring mental health and substance use disorder diagnoses. The facility included a secure medical detoxification program and 28 days of inpatient treatment. Clients would typically enter the detoxification building and spend three to six days under medical supervision. During their time in detox, many of them would have to address legal issues around an arrest or probation violation.

On discharge from detoxification, most were offered a referral to the 28-day inpatient treatment. Typically, they would attend court the morning of discharge and ask for a continuance so that they could attend inpatient treatment. Their discharge from the detox program was coordinated with one of the two days a week I facilitated a dual diagnosis group, so that they could attend their first group at the start of inpatient treatment. Each group was two-and-a-half hours, two days a week for a total of five hours of group per week.

It was clear to me that some—maybe most—of the clients entering my group were "coerced" into selecting treatment: "Do you want to go to jail today, or do you want to stay here and go into treatment?" Still, it is important to keep in mind that they had a choice and selected treatment. Most, if not all, of the clients that were referred from detox had a long history of addiction, mental health issues, and behavioral health and addiction treatment, including individual and group therapy.

The dual diagnosis groups were open-ended, meaning that new clients entered as clients who had completed 28 days in treatment were discharged. As a result, we had a core population who were familiar with our group process. In addition to attending group twice a week, each client had an addiction counselor who was responsible for testing, individual counseling, and discharge planning. Clients also had access to a psychiatrist for evaluation and medications if needed. Our population was not new to treatment programming. Most in-patient program clients had attended both inpatient and outpatient dual diagnosis process groups in the past, as well as AA and Narcotics Anonymous.

Clients would enter group feeling like a failure after a drug or alcohol "runner" and arrest, with the expectation that this was just another treatment experience. Their impression was that they needed to talk about their weaknesses and problems, admit to being powerless, receive critical feedback or confrontation from group members, talk about their worthlessness and bad decision making, stay with the program, and follow the 12 steps. My expectations and ideas for the group were very different.

I had learned from clients over the years in many settings that my group had to be "different" if I was going to be helpful. I needed to facilitate a therapeutic atmosphere of hope and join with clients to support them to become "customers" of therapy and change.

Notice that I do not go into the full SFBT process language and questions at the very start. That will come later in the group process. This intake is to orient the client and begin to build hope. I do not want to support the all-too-common idea that many mandated clients take with them into first day of treatment: "If I just comply and do my time here ..." It quickly becomes clear to those attending the group that the expectation is for them to do self-work and take responsibility for addressing whatever they have identified as problems.

Johnny entered the group after five days in detoxification, head down and avoiding eye contact, looking pale, body rigid and stressed. His marriage was in jeopardy; he had lost his job; and he had been arrested and charged as an accessory to grand theft auto and evading a police officer, among other things. He felt physically sick and weak, but he believed that he had to present as tough and confident.

Saul: Good morning. We have a new member today. Would you please introduce yourself?

Johnny: Johnny.

Saul: Hi, Johnny. Welcome to the group. Our group is for solution building and understanding. We want to create an environment of hope and confidence that will help you to figure out what you really want and how to get there. I know you've probably been through a lot recently, but I would bet that you are more than that—that you have a lot of strengths and helpful life experiences. We want to get to know you a little bit. Tell us a little about yourself.

Johnny: [Repositioning himself in his chair, sitting up, then leaning slightly forward and opening his eyes wide, he begins speaking very fast] Oh man, I can't believe it. I don't believe I'm here. I should have known it. Two months ago, I relapsed after an argument with my wife. She moved out and I just started drinking every day. She took the kids and moved in with her sister, so I said, "Screw it." Last week I was walking from home to the 7-11 and suddenly there he was on the corner—Jim, my old friend. Haven't seen him for more than a year, when he pissed off my wife and she told him to get lost. We partied a lot a few years ago. He's almost a brother to me but bad news. I said, "What are you doing here?" He points to a cherry candy apple red '63 Chevy parked on the street and says: "Hey man, look ... 409 ... I'm going to get one of those ... I was just at my girl's place down the block ... Walking to the 7-11 ... Come on, let's get a beer and catch up." This time I didn't say "no" to him.

Saul: What else can you tell us about yourself?

Johnny: I should have known better. We went to the 7-11 and bought two six-packs. We took the beer to my apartment and finished them quickly, talked about old stuff, and went back to get another six-pack. On the way back Jim asked me for a wire clothes hanger and then said: "Let's go for a ride." He jimmied the 63 Chevy's door open and hotwired the car. We were off. He was speeding, got on the highway going 80, 90, 100, and there were cops behind us. There were lights and sirens from four cop cars, then we began to skid sideways, hit the shoulder and slid into the grass, up the hill ...

Saul: Whoa, just a minute. I've heard a lot of "war stories" like this over and over during the past 30 years. That isn't what I'm interested in. I guess that I needed to ask the question in a different way. Johnny, tell me: what was the longest time you've been clean and sober?

Johnny: Two years, eight months, and seven days.

Saul: Wow, that's quite an achievement ... More than two-and-a-half years—almost three. How'd you do that? What helped?

Johnny: Well, I guess I really took care of my marriage and my kids— now she won't even talk to me, and I miss my kids. I went to work and liked my job, and the boss was a real good guy. Had a great sponsor, Bill; yes, he really helped. I did carpentry and built a lot of our furniture. Went to counseling with my wife, for our relationship and sobriety, and that was really good stuff until we got lazy about working on ourselves. I was attending three or four AA meetings a week and took night classes and job training for advancement. I was careful, only had sober friends, and mostly stayed away from old friends like Jim. We lived in a nice apartment that had a workout room and I would work out—sorry that I stopped. Oh, and I read good books with my wife instead of television—I think that helped us to be closer. We also ate healthier and went to church. I think that's what helped.

Saul: Wow, that's great stuff. I'm writing down everything so that you'll have a record of what has worked for you. Is there any-thing else that you can think of?

Johnny: Umm ... Oh yeah, I watched over my kid brother and helped him with school stuff. And another thing: I was journaling—you know, writing stuff down every night. I think that helped me to keep a perspective.

Saul: You're a lot smarter now. So, looking back, if you were to go home today, what else would you put into your recovery plan that would make success more likely—maybe the things that would have kept you from relapsing when you did?

Johnny: I think not gambling. I was doing it on the sly. I needed to be standing up for my family. Put them first. I wish I had. I was respecting my family by saying "no" to hanging out with Jim after my wife had it out with him. I could have been praying more and believing in myself, knowing I was worth it again like I used to. Probably not letting resentments get to me and talking honestly about them. I need to face up to my family stuff, I guess. It was stupid to think that I had it made and could have just a few beers with Jim. Maybe I will need to find a stress program. And I guess really being honest with my wife. I need to get her back, really badly. And I know that I'll need to do 90 meetings in 90 days like I did when I started in recovery.

I continued to write down everything he said.

Saul: Congratulations—you've gotten off to a good start writing the treatment portion of your discharge plan. Yes, that is what you've just done. If it's okay with you, I'm going to give this list to your counselor so he can put it in your file. Now you can focus on treatment here, and on whatever you need to do to get to discharge! Your discharge plan is pretty much outlined because of your good work today!

You could see change in Johnny's demeanor and hear it in his voice. Hope and motivation had been restored. He had likely become a willing client and perhaps had begun to build some confidence about his future. Johnny entered group expecting to get beat up emotionally, but instead we focused on strengths and solutions. He accomplished something meaningful the first day. It was not what he expected.

Johnny was off to a good start, becoming a customer of therapy. He had built a foundation for goals and had formulated at least a partial version of what he could do to restore some of what he had lost. I knew what had been helpful to him and what was important to him. I could become an advocate for him and talk about "what works" with his counselor. I knew some things about his "agenda," such as restoring his relationship with his wife and children; and I knew what to follow up with to learn about other parts of his "agenda." I also had a partial history that I could explore with him while he was a group member.

Years later, I ran into Johnny, his wife, and his teenage children, coming out of a restaurant. He hugged me! I complimented him on his beautiful family and told him that I could see what he fought for—they were worth all his hard work and sacrifice. He thanked me again and said that his first day in my group had helped him to turn the corner after he had given up on himself. He asked me to promise that if I ever wrote a book, I would include his story to help inspire others.

"I Would Bet That You Are More Than That"

You might have noticed that, after an introduction, my first question to Johnny was worded:

> I know you've probably been through a lot recently, but I would bet that you are more than that—that you have a lot of strengths and helpful life experiences. We want to get to know you a little bit. Tell us a little about yourself.

I have learned to include the phrase "I would bet that you are more than that" because I recognize that when a client is referred, we only get to see a snapshot that is more about the recent problem than the client's life. It is imperative to avoid judgments and clinical decisions until after we have learned about our clients. In addition, clients do not need to get beat up in therapy; they enter stressed and often beating up on themselves, and until we can relieve some of that self-inflicted trauma, it will be challenging for them to make substantive progress.

Group work will fundamentally resemble solution process. After discussing problems, and then acknowledging a client's circumstances, I have found that eliciting exceptions and solutions is the most prudent course. I am less interested in talking at length about the problem and instead will steer the discussion toward exceptions (when they are not doing the problem and instead doing at least part of the solution). Questions to inquire about how each client has already been doing part of the solution might sound like: "When have you wanted to drink but didn't? How did you resist? What helped?" Clients will hear themselves describing "what they need to do more of" to make the changes they desire. We need to be aware that our clients have talked the problem to death in AA and various treatment programs, so they clearly understand their vulnerabilities and weaknesses.

My interventions are crafted to build hope, willingness to put forth effort, and confidence in their strengths. We need to be consistent in giving compliments as we elicit stories of client successes or when they offer sound ideas about solutions. In order to achieve outcomes desired by clients, it is critical that, in addition to a collaborative relationship, we make it crystal clear that we care enough to really listen, understand, and maintain positive regard and hope, while being committed to helping clients to identify and accomplish their agenda. To be successful, clients do not have to come to therapy "for the right reason"; they just need to have the right experience in therapy.

The Power of Normalizing, Externalizing, and Reframing

Some widely known but perhaps "not used often enough" strategies for helping clients to maintain hope are "normalizing," "externalizing," and "reframing." Clients sometimes find themselves shackled by labels or a diagnosis. Whenever practical, it is better to talk about specific behaviors rather than labels or a diagnosis. "Self-esteem" is too vague a label to process with clients, so it might be better described for a particular client as "being able to confidently present your ideas in front of your class." "Codependency" might be more manageable as "giving away too much at your own expense."

If a client insists on self-describing with a label, inquire with questions to elicit what the solution might look like. For example, we could ask: "When you have self-esteem, what will you be doing differently?" We want clients to talk about problems or difficult circumstances without labels because behavioral descriptions are more manageable and less threatening than labels. When clients see reductions in the frequency or intensity of unwanted behaviors, it can help them to feel empowered, and they will be more likely to notice when they are doing the solutions. Early in my training, it was helpful when I learned that problems are not pathology and how we define them makes a difference.

When challenges or hiccups occur, normalizing can be a means to help clients stay on track. For example, after communicating a clear understanding of a father's explanation of a problem, we might normalize by saying:

> Many families suffer challenges like that—and it can be really overwhelming and difficult at times—but I can see that this is not the whole story. You're more than that! I want to hear about times when you have overcome problems like this one.

Follow-up questions to identify exceptions and solutions might include: "Tell me about times when this problem has been less burdensome or not happening?" Followed by a sequence that includes: "So how

Building a Positive, Hopeful Start 63

will you be doing more of that?" Then I take the opportunity to spend considerable time exploring with the family what is going well and give them compliments.

Externalizing is another strategy to address the client's perception of a barrier that is challenging the resolution of problems. We could externalize by asking, "The problem is out there; but you are the expert on your family, so tell me about a day when you kept it off your back"; or, "I can hear that this problem is a thorn in your side—so what have you been doing to get it out? What has worked well? How did you know to do that? What else will you be doing?"

Externalizing, normalizing, and reframing can work well in most cases. In reframing and normalizing, we might call what a person thinks by a different name, but we are careful not to contradict the client's reality. The idea is to expand a client's possibilities and diffuse the difficulty or hopelessness of the perceived problem. Making the problem smaller or manageable in symbolic ways can be immeasurably helpful to clients who feel burdened, overwhelmed, or powerless. We need to pay attention to the client's receptiveness and acceptance of our intervention and let them teach us what works for them.

Ten-Year-Old Billy

Sometimes it is helpful to disarm the problem by visualizing it as a benign object in order to defuse its perceived power. I was working with a family who had a ten-year-old son, Billy. He was struggling with a problem that made his stomach "hurt." Billy told us that the other kids at his new school did not like him and whenever he thought about it, he felt pain in his stomach. We were addressing the issue with him, and his parents were very helpful; but he continued to feel stomach pains. Billy sometimes held or rubbed his stomach during therapy. His parents had taken him to a physician, and he had several medical tests, all of which were within normal limits, so we were relatively certain that there was no medical basis for his pain.

During the second session, I noticed that Billy had taken a small rock out of his pocket and held it in his hand, close to his stomach. When I asked him about it, he told me that he had picked up the rock near his house the day his family entered therapy. Billy continued to hold the rock throughout the session, and I noticed that he fidgeted with it whenever he talked about school. Toward the end of one of the sessions, I said, "Billy, put your problem—the one about not having friends at school—in the rock and continue to carry it around with you in your pocket every day."

Billy reported during the next session that he no longer had stomach pain but hated that he had to carry the rock around. During the next two sessions, Billy continued to report that he no longer felt stomach pain. In the session that followed, he told me that he had been sitting with three other students at lunch and they had been friendly toward him. His parents reported that they had gotten him into Scouts and Little League practice had begun. I noticed that Billy had not taken the rock out of his pocket during the session and asked him about it. He told me that he had thrown the rock into the field near his house and did not need it anymore.

Assessments Are Interventions

Assessment evaluators and clinical report writers have a critical role in defining the problem and building hope. Too often, treatment gets off on the wrong foot because of indifference, stereotyping, or lack of sensitivity by report writers. Clients often enter therapy feeling defeated and defensive after reading about themselves. I would advocate for reports to reflect strengths, opportunities for change, and input from the client themselves about what they need. Clients and agencies need to share ownership and their ideas need to have equal input throughout the written document. When a family's ideas are put under a subsection named something akin to "Family's view of the problem," it can appear as if the case manager or clinician is saying, "Here's what the 'in denial' or 'lying' family says."

A single-parent family was referred for therapy to address parenting issues and child behavioral issues. Tom was a 15-year-old whose mother had reported him as "incorrigible" and uncooperative with chores. She complained to the school, the juvenile justice authorities, and state Mental Health, asking for help. Eventually, she locked her son out of the house and told him that she was tired of his messiness and uncaring attitude. He went to school the next morning looking disheveled from spending the night sleeping in his backyard, without a shower or change of clothes. The school called Child Welfare and mom told them that she knew he had friends, and the weather was warm, so he would not be in danger. When pressed, she admitted that if he had come to the door that night and asked, she would have let him back in the house.

We had an initial meeting with Tom and his mother. It was clear that Tom was embarrassed and hurt, yet he professed love for his mother and regret that things had gotten so out of control. He asked for help, and I could see that Tom would be a customer in therapy for resolution with his mother; but he did not want to hear it was his fault. Mom presented as a complainant. I could hear her frustrations and how several years of parenting a teen had worn her down. Mom said she feared losing her son to foster care, so I assured her that I would be an advocate and would do everything I could to ensure that did not happen. Admittedly, in addition to fear, she was feeling hopeless and angry, and she brought with her the report for the court that the Child Welfare evaluator had given her for review. Mom referred to the report and wanted me to explain to Tom that this was his fault and things were really serious. The first page contained a "Summary for the Court":

> Tom is a 15-year-old who is oppositional-defiant. His mother complains that anything she asks him to do is met with resistance. She states that the only things he cares about are his friends and getting his driver's license. She regrets that she promised him that he could get a driver's license if he had a B average because he is a B+ student. His room is messy, and mother has too much to do to keep the house clean by herself.

In the meeting, I used reflective listening to validate the feelings of both mom and Tom, and I explored with them exceptions to the current difficulties. There were many examples of times when they had cooperated and resolved their issues without outside help. There was more than a week remaining before the court report had to be formally submitted, so I had some time to intervene. I secured permission from Tom and his mom for us to meet with the Child Welfare evaluator and ask her to consider rewriting the court report to reflect a more accurate picture of them. When we met with the Child Welfare evaluator, she insisted that the facts in the report needed to remain intact, but she agreed that an accurate characterization was important. We rewrote a portion of the report without changing any of the facts, and the newly edited report went to the judge. The first-page summary was changed to read as follows:

> Tom is a 15-year-old who lives with his mother. He is a B+ student, has several good friends, and is socially active. Mother has shown effectiveness as a parent by supporting his educational efforts and offering Tom the opportunity to get a driver's license as long as his grades average at least a B. She has found it difficult, however, to get him to comply with chores at home and keep his bedroom clean. Her concern is twofold: she needs help around the house, and she wants to teach him responsibility. Tom has not been motivated to cooperate with her requests. In order to secure the cooperation of 15-year-olds who are individuating, it is often helpful for them to understand the reasons for a parent's requests and then be given an incentive to cooperate. Mom and Tom have already shown they can facilitate an arrangement of cooperation for rewards.

Without objection from the case manager or Child Welfare, the court declined to continue the agency's jurisdiction and closed the case, but recommended that Tom and his mom continue in therapy. They were motivated to continue counseling, and things had already improved greatly between them.

Mom became a customer of therapy and supported her son's efforts in school. The newly written report gave them both hope and started them on a path of greater cooperation and consideration. It was not a surprise that they worked out a plan where mom gave Tom an allowance contingent on his cooperation with chores and keeping his room clean. He got his driver's license and was allowed to use her car as long as he paid for gas—which he paid for using his allowance for completing chores. The information in the revised report summary on the first page provided everything they needed to figure out a workable solution. They had their solution from the beginning but, as often occurs, did not realize it.

Non-blaming, strength-based writing leads to a greater understanding of intent and helps clients find solutions that work for them. We want to represent all views in ways that engage and empower, rather than alienate clients or triangulate them. Reports and assessments are in themselves clinical interventions that affect outcomes, positively or negatively. Collaborative report writing with the family as a partner provides the writer opportunities to identify the family history and culture, family strengths, what has worked in the past, what resources are available, and the family's history of problem solving. Beyond the basic assessment information and writing functions, the assessment interview can help the family to build hope and confidence, identify potential solutions, and be motivated to participate in treatment.

"Put Your Problem in That Chair"

Over the years, I used the Gestalt "empty chair" concept with clients who came to therapy with partner issues when their significant other was unwilling to attend. Although not actually couple's counseling, those clients benefited from a discussion with their "partner," who was represented by the chair. Then the client was asked to "switch" chairs to become the partner in the conversation, so I could see the relationship dynamics and dialog as represented by my client. This was a helpful tool for me to better understand and assess the situation. Clients often felt empowered and validated, and usually reported greater understanding—even forgiveness. I have used the empty chair for a client's talk with a parent, a boss, or even a deceased person as part of the solution process.

Several clients who grew up in families with a parent who was addicted, and perhaps abusive, had read books that discussed the "inner child." They had become actively invested in "inner child work." Inner child work is a self-care concept that involves symbolically holding and talking to the "child you were," who lives internally as part of you, burdened with unresolved issues and hurts. Clients who practiced inner child work were able to take the feelings and burdens inside them, which had been elusive, and ultimately process resolution through self-talk and self-care. Clients reported feeling empowered rather than powerless. Whether through an empty chair or inner child work, clients felt more control and power when they were able to move the "problem" from inside themselves to outside themselves, symbolically. Inner child work is described in depth in Chapter 9.

A young, insightful woman named Kathy was referred to me and inspired an intervention that merged solution process, strategic ideas, and an "empty chair." She had previously been in treatment with four psychologists—one about five years prior and the other three over the previous two years—and she was feeling desperate: "I don't want to be here. I hate therapy and I'm not good at it." Kathy was experiencing panic attacks and was having them at work. Her manager had sent her to the company's employee assistance program (EAP), which contacted their insurance company's "managed care program" for one last referral. It was clear to Kathy that this was pretty much her last chance to keep her job.

Kathy was feeling hopeless when she arrived for the first appointment, and tearfully told me of the problems at work that had come about as a result of her panic attacks. She reported that in the past year she had been overcome at a business meeting, in her office, and at a staff meeting. She disclosed a history of panic attacks beginning when she was 16 years old. The frequency and intensity had accelerated over the previous five years. Kathy shared that since adolescence, she had seen physicians, psychologists, and an EAP clinical social worker. "Nothing helped to stop the demons from attacking me," she said. "They have too much power over me. How can I stop them?" I could literally see the powerlessness and desperation on her face and in her body language.

I asked her exception questions to learn about times when she did not have panic attacks, when they were less intense, or when they did not last as long. Kathy alluded to being through this process before, without resolution. "Each one is ugly, and I don't have any control. Some are stronger. It's like a demon possesses me." She remembered several panic attacks in detail and became livid as she described how they had consumed her. I said, "It sounds like the panic attack is, as you said, like a 'demon.'" She responded, "I wish that demon was right here so I could take it by the neck and choke it to death. But it's inside me. It lives inside me. I can't do anything to stop it. It is invisible. It controls me."

I knew that whatever the intervention, it had to be different for her than previous ones. Every attempt by professionals to intervene had failed her. Kathy needed hope; and as long as the panic attacks were inside her and unpredictable, she said she would feel powerless and hopeless. So, guided by her words, I borrowed a page from a strategic task and merged the Gestalt empty chair with client-need-driven solution ideas to help her manage "the problem." After all, she had told me what she needed; and I could see a way for her to set the stage to take action.

How a client defines the problem and solution is the key to creating a deliberate exception. Kathy needed a meaningful exception to the power-lessness and hopelessness she felt—an exception that would put her in control, and that she could build on. I said, "You know, Kathy, it's clear to me from what you've said that the panic attacks alone are not really the problem." Her eyes widened, and she asked, "What do you mean?" I replied:

> You're here because you are having the panic attacks at work. You said that you rarely have them at home; and when you do, you said they do not last long and are not a big deal. You described the idea of having them at home as you "couldn't care less." Can you see that the panic attacks aren't so much the problem as the timing of the panic attacks? It's about when and where you have them.

Kathy became very interested and asked, "What do I need to do, then? Have them only at home?" We both laughed, but I could see her processing the idea. I waited several seconds and then answered:

> Yes. If it might help your situation at work, are you interested in scheduling panic attacks at home, several days a week, at a time that is convenient for you? We can talk more about the details and your goal to get more control over that panic attack demon. Perhaps you could practice how you might do it. Are there days and times convenient for you to force yourself to have a panic attack at home?

Kathy initially picked three weekdays at 7:00 p.m. I elicited from her a plan. She offered to sit on the chair in her bedroom, use a folding chair to represent the panic attack, and coax the panic attack to begin "right then and there." I gave her only a very general outline of what she might do, leaving the most intricate details and words to her imagination. "Kathy," I said, "we're now going to practice how you can take charge and get control of the panic attack." "Okay," she shrugged. "So, what do I do?"

> Well, Kathy, you know a lot about the panic attacks. I suppose you can go ahead and do what you said you wanted to do. Take control and tell the panic attack what you think of it, and what you want. You want to be the one to decide when to have a panic attack.

I moved a chair in front of Kathy and said, "Here it is. Talk to it." "Really?" she asked. I replied, "Absolutely—here it is, right in front of you. Tell that panic attack 'demon' what you think of it, and then take control."

Kathy stared silently for a minute, and then became immersed in the role, sternly scolding the symbolic panic attack chair, getting firmer over time, and telling it that she was going to take control. I could see her confidence building and her resolve taking over. She began to delight in her newfound ability to strike out at the panic attack and she stood up, leaning over the panic attack chair and assertively explaining that she had had enough. At the end of the session, Kathy stood up straight and looked less burdened, but still serious. I scheduled our next meeting for six days later, telling her that I believed she would do well with her empty chair home task, but to remember that this process was new to her, and she would get more and more skilled at doing it over time.

We scaled her willingness and confidence to complete the task. "On a scale of 0-10, how willing are you to complete this task?" Kathy responded with a 10 and anchored her rating with, "I just have to do this. My job depends on it. I will write the days and time on my calendar to be sure." On the confidence scale, she also responded with a 10. "As I said," she explained, "I have to do this. When I promise to do something, I do it. Yes, confidence is a 10." (I prefer a 0-10 scale because very discouraged clients would sometimes say "0" when I said 1-10, so to sidestep that, I began using 0-10 and it has worked well).

I did not hear from Kathy until she arrived for our next appointment. She was energetic and excited as she entered the room, and she began speaking as soon as she sat down. "Thank you, thank you, thank you!" she said. "I sort of did it—part of it—and I was a little nervous; but it felt really good." I said, "Tell me all about it." Kathy shared:

> I set up the folding chair, and said, "You are the panic attack, and we need to talk." I talked to my panic attack and told it, "I am in charge from now on. I decide when you can come out and never at work." Then I waited, and nothing happened. And nothing happened at work this week, so that was good.

I waited for the other shoe to drop—to hear Kathy explain what she meant by, "I sort of did it." There was silence and then she talked briefly about her work issues and how she had handled them. I finally asked her, "So, what did you mean when you said, '… sort of did it?'" She replied:

> Oh—I'm sorry. I meant that I tried to have a panic attack at home this week. I tried all three days when I set up the chair, and I told it that now was the time, to go ahead and do it. But it wouldn't work. Is that okay?

I told her how impressed I was for the work she did, and then asked her for her impressions. Kathy replied, "I guess that maybe the panic attack demon was weaker than we had thought? Is that possible?" She then smiled and said, "Um, I guess that's good?" I complimented Kathy and scaled her on confidence and hope, anchoring her progress with specific changes she identified and asking fast-forward questions that represented moving up one number on each scale. I told her that she was courageous and creative— "a great combination of strengths that will help you to succeed."

I also introduced a "confidence in personal power" scale. On a 0-10 scale, Kathy said that she was a 4, which meant that she was able to stand up to her problems, confront the "demon," and take care of herself. "I have free will and I can do what I need to beat this," was her remark. She said a 5 would mean that she was continuing to keep the "demon" in check; and that she would slow down and have breakfast in the morning, instead of worrying about having a panic attack at work and losing her appetite.

Over the next several weeks, Kathy continued with the empty chair task at home in addition to our practice in the office. We transitioned to 20 to 30 minutes of talk about what was going well in her life that she didn't want to change, and then—only if she wanted to practice—about 10 minutes of empty chair work to reinforce what she was doing at home. Then several weeks later, Kathy began the session by reporting that the day before, at work, she had felt herself getting a little dizzy and shaky, overcome by that panic feeling she dreaded. "I told it to stop," she said. "That I was in charge; that it had to wait until we got home; and I really pushed hard. It stopped. I did it. When I got home, I almost got it to start, but it wasn't strong enough. I was so exhausted that I went to bed. It was the best night's sleep I've ever had. I even ate breakfast and felt great all through the next day."

She continued in-session work for several months, seeing me once every two to three weeks. Kathy reported two panic attacks—neither one at work—and we agreed that she had all of the tools she needed. Our work then focused on several other issues that she raised, and for each she was able to identify exceptions and quickly resolve them, citing solutions that were already happening some of the time. Kathy told me that life was good, and she was relieved. She also came to recognize that she was less vulnerable to having a panic attack when she had slept well the night before. Kathy expressed her revelation as irony: "So when I used to have trouble sleeping because I was worried about having panic attacks, it made me have more panic attacks. How stupid is that?"

Kathy's confidence on the personal power scale was a 7 and she was very satisfied with her progress. After we processed her description of the anchors that made her a 7, she concluded that the 7 was actually very close to a 10. We mutually agreed to discontinue our regular therapy meetings, with the option for her to schedule an appointment at any time she felt it necessary. I followed up with her 90 days later, as I do with all my clients, and she reported doing well. About a year later, Kathy referred a friend to me, so I learned that she was still employed at the same firm.

Kathy's story illustrates the importance of really listening to a client. Therapists need to listen closely and hear the client's definition of the problem. They need to hear exceptions. And they also need to hear more than exceptions. Clients often give clues about a process or tasks that can lead to possible solutions. They also sometimes modify tasks or only do a portion of a task, which I interpret as, "They know better about what they need or do not need." And sometimes, as in Kathy's case, a mutually agreed upon task to help with one issue will inadvertently resolve a second issue.

Kathy's early disclosure that the panic attacks were less impactful at home was actually an exception that provided us with possibilities for completing her agenda. Her agenda was to stop having panic attacks at work, because she did not want to risk losing her job. Her goal never was to eliminate them completely. Working with her to find a solution meant helping her find a strategy to take charge of the time and place that the panic attacks occurred. She also was able to resolve her difficulties falling and staying asleep, and then recognized that a good night's sleep could be preventative. At some future date, if she is motivated to eliminate all panic attacks, or identifies other issues, what she has already accomplished is a strong foundation. Kathy was satisfied for the time that her problem was sufficiently resolved.

Reference

De Shazer, S., and Dolan Y. (2021) *More than Miracles: The State of the Art of Solution Focused Brief Therapy*. Classic ed. New York: Routledge.

6 Reluctant or Mandated Clients
Skills to Turn Visitors into Customers

Clients involved in the court system or referred through coercion by a family member or employer can pose special challenges. Court referrals or other "coerced" referrals can be "beartraps" for the therapist or counselor. These clients usually present as visitors in therapy and even more often as visitors over the agenda of the referral source. It is not their idea to be in treatment. Clinicians need to maintain positive regard, and to recognize the potential for triangulation and conflict between what the client accepts and the agenda driven by the referral source. There are strategies that can allow us to be client-need driven and at the same time stay out of the line of fire while addressing the referral source's agenda.

Mandated or coerced clients come from a variety of sources. I've received client referrals from courts, jails, probation and parole officers, spouses, parents, mothers-in-law, employers, schools, employee assistance program/managed care professionals, case workers, case managers, attorneys, and others. The process is similar in each case: the client does not want to be there, but comes because they have something on the line—something that they do not want to lose, something that they are trying to avoid, or something that they want to gain. In the case of a minor, it could also be that the child is the "identified patient" in the family system and the parents are forcing attendance.

Mandated or coerced clients might consider that something needs to change—maybe not them—and welcome the referral as a chance to state their case; but most do not. Imagine being told you have a problem, but you strongly disagree; or you do not want to address it; or you do not think it is really you who has the problem, but that your freedom, or marriage, or health, or financial wellbeing depends on convincing someone else—and a "shrink" —that it is not your problem, or it is no longer a problem, or it never was a problem. You think that maybe there are "sides," and the therapist is on the side of the referral source. You want to say that you do

DOI: 10.4324/9781003397380-6

not need to change, or that you are doing just fine. How difficult a place might that be for you?

Let's say that you had originally acknowledged a problem that needed to be corrected; and that to keep your freedom, or get your children back, or keep your job, you attended therapy. Listening to the directives of the medical and mental health professionals and a case manager, or a probation officer, or a teacher, or a judge, you cooperated and worked hard. You did everything that was asked of you. You met all your obligations and were given a clean bill of health, and the therapist signed off on a release from mandated therapy and counseling. Life is moving along more smoothly than ever; but then, instead of "case dismissed" as was promised, you are told that you will be receiving a revised case plan to complete. Maybe the agency is not confident about you; or perhaps your case has been transferred to a new case manager, or probation officer, or judge.

You are directed to reenter treatment—justified by some new but vague reason, or a lack of trust in your progress. You just want to go on and continue to work, to parent, to drive, or whatever. You know that you can handle life's challenges and the precipitating problem will not happen again. You did what was asked and now you want the system to leave you alone. But nobody is listening or acknowledging what you are saying, and you are mandated to attend therapy and other programming again. How difficult might that be to accept?

Now think about the therapist who receives the referral. They are given a snapshot of your life—not a video of your whole life and who you are—and told that you are court ordered, or required by a case plan, or somehow otherwise mandated to attend in order to keep your children, or stay married, or keep your freedom, or keep your job. When you attend the first meeting with the therapist and begin with, "I don't really belong here," or "I don't know why I'm here," or "I don't have a problem," or "I already addressed these things and I don't need more therapy," or "My parole officer has it in for me," or "This isn't fair," what impression will the therapist likely get about you as a client?

Trusting a therapist with your most sensitive emotions and secrets will be uncomfortable—even embarrassing and challenging. It can be especially difficult to admit to wrongdoing that put your children, your family, a pedestrian, or society in jeopardy. Certainly, it can be challenging to convince a therapist—and perhaps even more difficult to convince a public authority—that you are no longer at risk of making a similar error. Even if the most ideal circumstances exist around the referral and the client accepts that changes need to be made, accepting full responsibility and admitting fault when there is involvement by the justice system would make anyone feel vulnerable. Self-protection and protection of family will strongly play against full disclosure in many instances.

These are all real examples of what I have seen time and time again. Too often, things get off to a bad start unnecessarily. It is our professional and ethical responsibility to develop a collaborative therapeutic alliance with our clients regardless of the reason for referral or their initial willingness to cooperate. Clients have demonstrated that their demeanor, presentation, and characterizations at the start of therapy can potentially create a misunderstanding and "expectancy bias" that will negatively impact the course of therapy. A rule of thumb at some point in my career became, "Clients need to be given more than one chance to make a first impression."

Intake Processes Matter

We need to create a collaborative therapeutic alliance and atmosphere through genuineness, compassion, open-mindedness, and empathy. Our process needs to begin with an honest understanding of our client and their circumstances. Early on in the first session, we need to know "what and who is important to our client"; and the answers to the questions, "What needs to happen for you to say our time together was worthwhile?" and "How will you know when you don't have to come here anymore?" We can smooth things out a little by building hope, confidence, and willingness from the start with client strength compliments, positive expectations, and language that presupposes success. Ideas about resistance or denial will only sabotage the opportunity to engage the client in the therapeutic process.

As with any client, we begin with an intake that includes a thorough history and a cultural assessment. I have learned that with mandated clients, it is critical to develop an individualized and very detailed "informed consent" agreement that reflects my legal reporting responsibilities; the client's rights to privacy and confidentiality; a list of protections that clearly states I am committed to the client's wellbeing and success; obligations under the Health Insurance Portability and Accountability Act, 42 Code of Federal Regulations Part 2, and any other provisions regarding privacy and confidentiality; mandatory reporting requirements; and an acknowledgment of the referral source's purpose in directing treatment. Clients need to understand that I am a treatment provider for them and their family, not for the referring agency.

Clients have shown me that until I know the particulars of the referral, including who has a vested interest in the therapy, it is difficult to understand the client's concerns and motivation. As part of the intake process, which can take more than one meeting, I ask a series of questions that acknowledge and respect the perception, point of view, and ideas of the client. The original question sequence for mandated clients—which Insoo Kim Berg shared as part of a training I attended—reflects her philosophy and ideas as they are explained in *Interviewing for Solutions* by Peter De Jong and Insoo Kim Berg (2013, pp. 209-220). Powerful and constructive, I have found her approach to be invaluable in building a foundation for a collaborative therapeutic relationship. I have since made some modifications to the mandated client question sequence that reflects my experience with clients who arrive as "visitors" sent to therapy by a third party that wants them to change. Keep in mind that it is important to elicit from the mandated client what they view as the "payoff" for successfully completing therapy. Sequences can be individualized to fit for the client, but essentially, I will ask the following questions:

- "Whose idea was it for you to come here to see me?"
- "What makes _____ think you need to come for therapy or counseling?"
- "What does _____ think is the reason or cause of the problem?"
- "What does _____ have to see or believe to leave you alone?"
- "When was the last time you did those things or some of those things?"
- "What was different then?"
- "What did it take for you to do those things?"
- "What were some things that were helpful in getting you started?"
- "Who will notice first when you have completed the first step and then done some of these things?"
- "What will be different in your life when you've done some of those things?"
- "What difference will it make in your relationship with your family (your boss, your friends, your children)?"
- "What will they say you are doing different that you are not doing now?"
- "What will the payoff be for you?"

Words Matter: When to Separate from the Referral Source

To maintain trust and a collaborative therapeutic alliance, it is important for clients to know that I am not an arm of the court, case manager, or mother-in-law. How we phrase our questions can affect perception, trust, and behavior. If a client is going to trust me to work for them toward achieving their goals, reminding a client that "the judge has ordered ..." or "your case manager will not return your children if you ..." can be counterproductive. So, I "externalize" with questions such as the following:

- "What would the judge say about that idea?"
- "Do you think the judge would go for that?"
- "How would doing that affect your case manager's opinion?"
- "What would your mother-in-law do if you said that to her?"

Whenever possible, I want to use a client's words along with the language of hope, maintaining clear boundaries and avoiding judgment and triangulation. If we take a parental or authoritarian posture, we will sabotage cooperation and the potential for second-order change. It can be a balancing act, but externalizing or using metaphor can help to communicate without putting a client on the defensive. In all cases, we need to avoid a one-to-one conflict with our clients. An intern supervisor once told me, "When policy issues, laws or family are involved, stay out of the line of fire." The point is, if you never pick up your end of the rope, there is no tug of war!

During the therapeutic process and in co-constructing goals with our client, it is important to hear and use the client's "definition of the problem" and language, rather than strictly the terminology of the referral source. Mental Health, Child Welfare, the Department of Parole and Probation, the courts and various other agencies have their own technical language When clients are referred, probation agreements, court orders, case plans, or self-improvement plans identify with words how the entity defines the problem. So essentially, there can be two jargons in the spoken and written language: one from the client, which we primarily use with the client; and one that we include in reports or testimony to the referring authority. At the same time, the client might have a different version of what they need to do to satisfy the reason for referral or the purpose behind the need for behavioral change. We need to respect and satisfy our client's agenda while ensuring that the referral source's concerns are assuaged, and any mandates are satisfied. Straddling that line can be tricky.

Child and Family Teams

Families that are more on the "traditional" side with extended family supports have a level chance to fare well when referrals are made to competent social system agencies, whether child welfare, juvenile justice, mental health, or justice/family court. When agencies mandate a case plan or action plan for families that are non-traditional and/or have few natural family or professional resources, outcomes that leave the family intact and stronger are more challenging to achieve.

Socioeconomically disadvantaged families and families of color are at higher risk of losing custody or seeing their child incarcerated. In order to build a more level playing field while strengthening families and protecting children or vulnerable adults, during my tenure with Intensive Family Services (IFS) in the 1990s I promoted a process of child and family team meetings and facilitated "how to" workshops for professionals and family advocates. I would participate in live child and family team meetings to facilitate the process of planning, inviting, and holding meetings to iden-tify needs, resources, and solutions for families at risk.

Planning involves initially meeting with the client family and gathering as much information as possible about their strengths, resources, and goals. More often than not, there is important information that the super-vising agency does not have available in its records and perhaps has never known. My responsibilities begin with listening to the client-family and learning how they function, what their strengths are, and who their supports are. It is important to ask in-person questions of the client-family pertaining to who and what is important to them. Often it takes some prompting for them to think about people to invite. Questions that I have found to be helpful include the following:

- "If your car broke down, who would you call?"
- "If you needed groceries to feed your children, who could you depend on?"
- "If you came home to a medical emergency, who would you run to?"
- "If you were called into work unexpectedly and needed someone to watch your children, who would that person be?"
- "Who would you invite to your children's birthday party?"

Invitations to meetings need to include persons identified by the client-family as resources. In addition to professionals, advocates, and relatives whom the family might select, participants may include "fictive kin." Fictive kin are important "pseudo-family members" in many families—often more important than blood relatives but sadly not acknowledged or too often excluded as a resource by professionals and public agencies. They are more than supports or friends who help—they can be the closest "non-blood relatives" who children call "grandma," or "aunt," or "uncle." Fictive kin could include:

- the landlord who gives the children breakfast when mom has no eggs;
- the neighbor who watches the children while mom works and even shares her food stamps to help mom;
- the custodian who is mom's only source of transportation to child wel-fare appointments; or
- mom's lifelong friend who offers her a shoulder to cry on when things are tough.

I recall a meeting involving a young single mom with a history of sub-stance abuse and depression. Her three young children were about to be reunified with her after two years in foster care. Mom had complied with all the requirements of the court and case plan to get her children returned, but had a challenging history. As is common with addiction, at the beginning there were some bumps in the road. Mom overcame those difficulties and thrived, remaining sober and stable for more than 20 months.

In addition to completing each case plan item that was mandated, mom maintained a supervised visitation schedule to spend quality time with her children every week. The court had imposed certain conditions on her for reunification: continued sobriety with lab testing for verification; maintaining employment; providing shelter and support for her children; attending Narcotics Anonymous (NA) or Alcoholics Anonymous (AA) meetings; and weekly counseling. A child and family team meeting was called to put the reunification in motion, and if indicated, to physically return the children to their mother.

Mom was asked to identify family supports or advocates who could participate in the meeting, and initially was unsure whom to invite. Mom was the family scapegoat and did not have much family support. After some encouragement and questioning, she was able to identify her father's brother, Uncle Bob, who was also a scapegoat in his nuclear family; her church minister, who was involved at the local food bank and allowed AA and NA meetings to be held in his church; and a "fictive kin" neighbor who worked as a nurse's aide. There were more than ten other participants who attended the meeting, including a teacher; a Latchkey counselor; a Child Welfare supervisor; mom's licensed alcohol and drug counselor; a welfare worker; and an agency family services worker.

It is imperative to avoid a contentious meeting with an outcome driven solely by professionals or those with a bias toward the child, parents, or foster parents. Some participants may have their own agenda, driven by ideas other than the goal of identifying resources and strategies to ensure safety and nurturing while preserving the family. Oppositional alliances between professionals, caregivers, agency staff, teachers, family members, and advocates can contaminate and prejudice the outcome.

It is important to plan every part of the meeting in advance and have at least the following ready: a seating chart (you do not want "foes" to be sitting across from each other and making eye contact); a list of rules and protocols for politeness; and a written item agenda that includes introductions, a statement of the goal for the meeting, a discussion of strengths and challenges, documented changes that indicate progress or setbacks, family resources and supports in place, an explanation of issues or problems facing the family, a current plan and benchmarks, and next steps.

There was a high-powered alliance against this young mother at the meeting. Opposed to the reunification order were the Child Welfare case manager; the foster parents; the therapist from mom's pre-sobriety days; one of the children's teachers; and one of mom's sisters. The case manager and foster parents had met with and recruited the therapist from mom's pre-sobriety days, the older sister, and the teacher to partner with them at the meeting to offer a recommendation to slowly reunify the children over a couple of years by allowing overnight home visits with mom only two days a week.

In the meeting, the case manager strongly presented her concerns. The other contrarians also made their case against mom as a parent, based solely on her old history and speculation. Mom was barely holding up under the barrage of criticism. Seeing that mom was fragile and nervous, the case manager began to interrogate her in a scolding tone:

Case manager:	You're supposed to pick up your children from Latchkey by 5:30 Monday through Friday, right?
Mom:	Yes, of course—I'll pick them up after work, right from work. I get off at 5:00.
Case manager:	Well, I can't check on you every night at 5:30 to see if you have your children and are home for dinner. If I can't check, I can't trust that you're not off on some drunken runner somewhere. You have a history.
Mom:	Well, I'm not like that anymore. I wouldn't; you have to trust...
Minister:	[Interrupting] Excuse me ma'am. I see. You can't check to see if she picked up the children. Okay, well I can. I can be at their house at 5:30; or I can pick the kids up for her and be at her house for dinner every weekday evening if that would help. In fact, I will leave you a voicemail when I get to the house, so you'll know that the kids are home and I'm with them, and if their mom is here too.
Mom:	You'd do that? Thank you, thank you. [Mom begins to cry].
Case manager:	Fine. But that's only part of the problem. I have more than 30 families on my caseload, more than 60 kids. I can't check every week to see if she is going to NA and AA. I can't get anyone there to talk to me about attendance or progress anyway. I just want what is best for those children.
Uncle Bob:	Well, look—I have more than 30 years of sobriety and I've been a sponsor many times. I'm also a life coach. I attend meetings almost every day and help run them. How about if I let you know, if my niece will give me permission, each time I see her in attendance. In fact, I will take her to meetings if she's okay with it.

Mom:	Yes, of course. Yes, that would be great. Thank you. [Mom really is sobbing hard. It strikes me that likely no one has ever stood up for her in her whole life.]
Case manager:	And who will be watching the children when you are at meetings? Or counseling? You can't afford more childcare.
Neighbor:	The meetings are after work hours, yes? I can watch them anytime you need me after 5:00 p.m. In fact, I can sometimes watch them during the day on Fridays and Saturdays. I work four ten-hour days a week.
Uncle Bob:	We can work that out. Nice thing to do.
Neighbor:	And you can be sure I will fill in anytime you need me. We can all make this work. The kids will be well taken care of.
Case manager:	You can't just watch the kids. You have to be approved. I don't know you. Have you a drug history or ever been arrested?
Neighbor:	No. I work as a nurse's aide in the hospital. I can give you whatever references you want. Give me the paperwork.
Case manager:	I will. Okay then. This is for the children. I want everything in writing.

The result is that the team voted to support the reunification conditionally. Not only did mom have her children returned, but less than two years later she and the children were released from the jurisdiction of Child Welfare and the court. Without the advocacy and supports, the chance of reunification would have been slim. Knowing that almost all parents want a better life for their children, I can begin a constructive process—even in the most challenging cases—by asking, "What will you be doing to give your children a better life, and what might be helpful to you?"

Teaching Need Not Be Treacherous

At IFS, I was responsible for a program that provided in-home family therapy to families designated as high risk with few resources, at imminent risk of having their children placed into therapeutic foster care. A provision attached to our grant mandated that we include "parent training" as part of our list of service offerings. Eligibility for family services required that at least one parent had a mental health "Axis I" diagnosis in addition to a substance use diagnosis. Parents could decline services but then would risk at least temporary loss of physical custody with the potential for termination of parental rights, so there was coercion involved. These were families who primarily had and only knew to use corporal punishment, but now were court ordered not to use any form of physical discipline.

We offered families a free clinical assessment and a 30-day trial period to get to know us. Invariably, they embraced us and accepted in-home clinical services. Families appreciated our family- centered language and sincere concern for their wellbeing. We used solution-focused brief therapy in conjunction with innovative non-blaming solution-oriented methods, so as they made progress there were compliments. In contrast to months or even years of getting beat up by Child Welfare and the courts, their time with us felt safe and empowering. However, we knew that telling a parent how to parent their children would predictably be met with an under-lying attitude of, "Who do you think you are, telling me how to parent my kids?"

Our primarily role with the family was to provide therapy. It would have been fine to externalize the issue with, "The judge and your case man-ager ordered that you cannot spank your kids, so what are you going to do instead?" Parent training is psychoeducational and, on the surface, would conflict with the core philosophy of client-centered therapies. Telling a parent that there is a better way to talk to and discipline their children while maintaining a collaborative therapeutic atmosphere is challenging. But under the provisions of our grant, we were tasked with teaching "parenting" in a way that the parent would have a practical understanding of an alternative to using physical discipline.

"Timeouts" were one of the approved parenting strategies under the grant. Our guidelines said that we had to present parent training as non-blaming, constructive, and effective. Rather than merely bringing out the teaching kit and workbook, and going over it page by page, I found a way to use metaphor, based on a real-life experience. Here is how I explained timeouts to parents before giving them, for use as a reference, a workbook on how to use timeouts with their children:

> I have wonderful children and I'm a very proud parent. You know what it's like to love your children and want the best for them. I came across an idea for using "timeouts" when there were problems, and I first began using them with my son Jonathan when he was about two years old. The idea was for us to separate in order to calm things down and then discuss a solution to make things right. So, when Jonathan was about two, we started with a two-minute timeout; and as he got older, we increased the time we would separate a little bit each year or so. When he was about ten years old, we started doing ten-minute time outs. And we would try to do separation in a way where it was not a punishment but a time to think about what happened, then get together to correct whatever the problem was.

What we did was alternate who went to his room. For example, Jonathan would go to his room for the first timeout, and I would go to my room for the next one. It didn't matter who went where as long as we separated to think about things and what to do about them; but it worked great to alternate each time. It seemed fair and that helped with compliance. It helped avoid the possibility for defiance. You know what I mean—we don't need an argument while we're taking control as a parent and deciding what to do. The idea was to separate and calm down, not to punish—at least not yet.

Timeouts worked smooth as silk year after year. And then one day, when Jonathan had just turned 13, I came home, and he was sitting in the family room watching television. On the floor were his baseball glove, baseball, hat, cleats, bat, and sweatshirt. I said, "Jonathan, you know better. You have to put away your stuff before you watch TV or do anything else. Pick up your things." Jonathan said, "Dad, shhh, I'm watching TV. I'll pick them up later." So, I tried to ask again calmly, "Hey, you know the rules. You're lucky it's me who got home first. Mom would be pissed. Just pick up your things." Then he got louder and said, "Dad, please stop, I'll do it after my show. Not now."

I knew I couldn't stay calm too much longer, so I initiated a timeout by saying, "Okay, we need to take a timeout. It's your turn to go to your room. See you back here in ten minutes and we'll work this out." I expected the usual response: "Okay, Dad, okay"; but instead, Jonathan stood up, faced me, and looked me in the eyes. He had this mischievous look that I'd never seen before, and a wry smile. Then he turned around and walked out the front door, slamming it behind him. I was stunned; like most parents, my instinct was to go after him, grab him, and force him back into the house. But I stopped myself as I thought about the workshop that I had just happened to attend the day before.

I had attended a workshop on parenting called "The Illusion of Control." The premise of the workshop was that we never really have control of our children—only the illusion of control; and once we lose that illusion, we lose it forever. I began to pace. My thoughts were: "I am screwed—I'm going to lose control forever. He's only 13; crap, five more years of adolescence. Teenage years. What can I do? I need to do something. He needs to know I'm in control." I walked over to a window next to the front door and peeked outside. There was Jonathan, sitting on the curb, looking up toward the sky. I struggled with how to handle the situation, not knowing what to do. Then it struck me—and I knew what to do.

I slowly walked outside in the direction of where Jonathan was sitting, careful not to make any eye contact. Sitting next to him on the curb and looking up at the sky, I said, "Jonathan, you are amazing.

I am so impressed with you. You are so smart." He looked toward me, but I continued to avoid eye contact, instead looking up at the sky. I said, "It is such a beautiful day. Bright, warm sun; blue sky; cool breeze. What a great idea to take your timeout here, outdoors. You have about six minutes left. I'll see you in the family room then." And I stood up without making eye contact, turned around, and walked slowly into the house.

Several minutes later, Jonathan came back into the house and cautiously walked into the family room. "I'm sorry, Dad," he said. I said, "That's okay—let's pick your things up and put them away. I'll help." He hugged me and we picked up his baseball gear together. He never again challenged a timeout.

I like to present this rendition colorfully with some theater in my story-telling, and almost universally, parents find the story amusing. The idea to be non-blaming, consistent, and constructive is generally understood and well received. Most parents are willing, if not enthusiastic about trying timeouts; and with some coaching along the way, the teaching process is usually successful.

Reference

De Jong, P., and Berg, I. K. (2013). *Interviewing for Solutions*. 4th Ed. Belmont, CA: Brooks/Cole.

7 Dire Straits

Heroic Clients Who Overcame Powerful Headwinds

In 2001, I was invited to present a workshop at a conference sponsored by the University of Nevada, Las Vegas. The theme was about building hope and empowering clients who were feeling disempowered and hopeless. I began by introducing neurolinguistics and presupposition, and then gave examples of exception questions and coping questions that had worked well for my clients. I emphasized that we need to use the client's words to define the problem. Next, I discussed several case examples and made the statement that when I persist in a "there must be something" line of questioning, "hopeless" clients come around and reveal something that they are doing for which I can give a compliment. There was a murmur in the group of 90 attending my seminar, and one of the clinicians raised her hand. She told me that she had a client who was negative "all of the time" and she could not imagine getting her to say something that would warrant a compliment.

I asked her, "Are you familiar enough with your client to roleplay her with me?" She responded, "Yes, absolutely." I asked her to briefly fill me in about her client and she said, "My client is a single mom with two young girls, elementary school age." So, after settling on a fictitious name to use, we began the roleplay. Seven or eight exchanges into the dialoging, she held firm with statements such as, "I'm a terrible mother, lying in bed all morning, sometimes all day, not paying attention to my children. Life sucks. Nothing has ever gone well for me. Everything is awful. I'm barely getting by, hardly coping with anything." I responded sympathetically with an acknowledgment that things sounded really difficult, and then said, "I believe you that it has been challenging; but there must be some days, or maybe parts of a day, when things are better—just a little bit?" Her response was something like, "Never—every day is awful. I am a horrible person and a terrible mother." We continued our exchange, and I asked her exception questions such as, "Tell me about a time when you did something that was fun or nurturing for the kids." She sidestepped each question or responded negatively.

DOI: 10.4324/9781003397380-7

I was waiting for the right moment to ask a "coping question." My work with clients has taught me over the years that the words and the timing are critical. If I tried to intervene too much or too strongly, I would lose her to all the negativities. Asking to see a picture of the children and then commenting on how they look or how nicely they are dressed is sometimes a way to lighten the mood; but that option was not available to me in this roleplay. She continued her hopeless words with, "My children see my anguish and they have to live with me. They are great kids to put up with this." I followed up with reflective, clarifying statements as feedback: "I'm sure you love your children"; and "They are living with you despite your anguish." She acknowledged that she loved her children more than anything, which gave me an opening, so I said, "Things sound really awful at your house. Are your children malnourished and emaciated?"

Her response was immediate and firm: "No, they're not malnourished. I wouldn't let them starve. They are well fed and healthy!" Nodding my head, I hesitated a couple of seconds before responding with:

> They are not starving? You mean that with all your anguish, all the difficulties, as horrible as things seem, you find a way to feed your children, to keep them healthy; and then you found a way to get here today for our appointment. I'm impressed by how strong your love for them must be. How come things aren't worse? What is it about you that you can rise above your gloom to keep your children fed and healthy, and get up this morning and come to my office on time for today's appointment?

Of course, the attendees' attention and thirst for more ideas were clearly noticeable after that exchange. Twenty years later, I can still attest to the effectiveness of presupposition and coping questions with discouraged and disenfranchised clients. Presupposition can and should be introduced from the onset of therapy. Coping questions are more sensitive and timing is critical, necessitating a therapist's patience to follow the client's lead. With the proper use of neurolinguistic language and sensitivity to a client's readiness, I have found that even the most reluctant or "down-and-out" clients respond and thrive when we introduce coping questions as part of our intervention.

Presupposition, Coping Questions, and "Problem to Solution" Processing

Fighting back against the desperate reality of "nothing will get better" requires a heroic mentality and a willingness to take on what looks improbable, if not impossible. When clients are faced with a discouraging situation, presupposition and coping questions can be effective in challenging feelings of hopelessness, while at the same time helping the client to notice a measure of success that already exists. It is often the small things that the client does to keep things from getting worse. These small things are the first steps that the client needs to build on in order to succeed. Clients benefit when they are reminded of and encouraged to continue to use their coping skills. At Intensive Family Services (IFS), we noticed how even the faint possibility of hope coupled with a small dose of change in the client and the system opened the floodgates to significant progress. (Chapter 11 talks about IFS families as families with challenges and few resources.)

Therapists can be a catalyst for desired change when they open the door for clients to describe what the change will look like and how the change will happen. We can teach clients, through the phrasing we choose, to think of positive change as inevitable and problems as transient. In presupposition, we use "definitive statements" to represent that desired change will happen, and "possibility statements" to imply that problems are less likely to reoccur. Neurolinguistics is a powerful piece in "problem to solution" processing, goal setting, and fast-forward questioning.

Definitive statements represent something a client wants to happen and are constructed using the word "when"; changing the tense; using qualifiers of time or intensity; adding terms such as "yet" or "so far"; or restating a problem as a goal. Examples might include the following:

- "<u>When</u> things are better, who will notice first?"
- "<u>When</u> you are able to tell her what you want, what exactly will you say?"
- "You haven't gotten much understanding <u>yet</u>. So, what will you notice first …?"
- "Your efforts haven't been recognized <u>so far.</u>" When they are recognized …"
- [Client complains that no one will hire him] "Oh, so you want to find a job …?"

Possibility statements imply "if" a problem were to happen again, the client would know how to handle it. Generally, the word "if" is used in conjunction with a question about how the client will handle the problem now that they are better equipped to deal with it. Examples might include the following:

- "<u>If</u> it were to happen again, what would you do differently this time?"
- "With everything you know now, and all your strength and resolve to make this marriage work, if that were to happen again, how would you handle it?"

Coping questions are used when other methods have not provided exceptions or when a client indicates hopelessness. Coping questions are sometimes regarded as the "last resort" for disparaged clients. When coping questions are used properly and appropriately followed by compliments, they can initiate a process that increases client participation and hope. Examples might include the following:

- "How come things aren't worse?" Followed up with a sequence of questions such as, "Wow, despite your [client's words], you decided to move ahead; how did you find the strength to do that?"
- "What is it about you that you survived?"
- "How did you cope with that?"
- "How did you find the will to do that?"

My favorite coping question is, "How come things aren't worse?" It is not unusual for clients to look at me with surprise, which might be their way of communicating, "How could you ask me a question like that?" A client once said, after she answered the question and we did some processing, "Were you blaming me for not doing worse?" I answered, "That's exactly what I was doing. It is about you having the strength and will to cope and then move forward regardless of how difficult things may get. I was confident that you had everything you needed."

Examples of compliments that can be given after a positive client experience with a coping question could include the following:

- "I'm really impressed by your survival skills."
- "You must have a strong will to succeed."
- "You must really love your children."

Compliments are an integral part of strength-based discussions. Solution therapists fuel the "problem to solution" process by following up compliments with "How did you do that?" inquiries coupled with fast-forward questions, such as "What will happen next that will indicate you're on track?" When used strategically and appropriately, compliments can solidify progress and motivate a client to continue constructive efforts. On the other hand, if formulated improperly or not genuine, compliments can sound hollow and be a minefield for the therapeutic relationship. Generally, we want to avoid compliments unrelated to progress or effort, such as "You look nice today."

Therapeutic compliments are meaningful and acknowledge real progress or strengths related to a client's agenda or goals (de Jong & Berg 2013, pp. 122-125). As you will read in the case example that follows, an exchange that features compliments might begin with, "What will happen next that will tell you that you're on track to putting this con-flict behind you and improving your relationship with your coworkers?" Your client answers, "I would make a better effort to be more of a team player—maybe by offering to help load their trucks if I've already finished loading mine." Then, during the next appointment, you ask your client what was different at work that week, and your client says, "A couple of my coworkers took me to lunch." You ask, "Oh, what prompted them to take you to lunch?" Your client says, "I guess they were thankful that I helped them load packages." The follow-up and compliment might be:

> You said that the next sign of being on track was that you would offer to help coworkers. That's impressive—even courageous—that you helped after all the strife you have experienced at work. And they took you to lunch! I want to hear more about what happened at lunch; but first I want to understand how you decided to help them load packages and how you put that hurtful incident last month behind you.

Presupposition, coping questions, and "problem to solution" processing are discussed in Appendix F.

Angie: "Life Should be Enjoyable"

Reflecting on my clients and the issues they brought to therapy, many women in their mid 20s to late 30s who had suffered emotional, physical, or sexual abuse as children found themselves hitting an emotional wall that prompted them to attend therapy. They had been adept at compartmen-talizing and were self-supporting, appearing confident and strong, until the emotions from a history of trauma caught up with them. Their strong work ethic and avoidance of deep, long-term emotional connections might have appeared to others as strength and independence. Commonly, they hid their trauma—or at least its severity—from acquaintances, friends, and coworkers.

Literally, I had dozens of clients who would have fitted that descrip-tion. Their survival skills, refined over years of coping, allowed them to appear functional and avoid being vulnerable to other people. They had lost sight of their strengths and did not recognize that they possessed skills that could help them address their childhood trauma and heal. Their well-guarded secret was that they believed they were defective. I knew how to be helpful as a therapist; but I also had to be aware of the potential for transference, especially with clients who had been groomed and abused by male relatives.

After several years of what might appear from the outside as a somewhat mundane adult life, trauma can emerge as hopelessness and desperation, or a loss of confidence. One of my clients, Angie, stands out in my memory, and I have used parts of her story in workshops and intern training seminars over the years. As is often the case for those who suffered through a dysfunctional family and childhood trauma, Angie's first ten years of adulthood looked from the outside to be quiet and uneventful. Her defenses were sophisticated, and she was able to keep herself together emotionally with a little help from distractions such as work, interests that did not include intimacy, and using alcohol as a sleep aide. Eventually, Angie recognized that she deserved better; but the first few meetings with her were characterized by feelings of hopelessness and despair.

The precipitating incident that brought her to therapy involved a frustrating Friday evening. Following a very hectic 12-hour workday, she was looking forward to cooking herself an extra-nice dinner at home. Angie was just finishing cleaning up after dinner when she noticed a water leak under the kitchen sink. She had tools and knew enough about plumbing to at least attempt a temporary repair; but the repair turned out more complicated than she had anticipated, and took her more than an hour to complete. A short time later, with the dishwasher running, a worse leak occurred, and it took every towel she had to dry the floor and cabinet under the sink. Exhausted, she sat on the kitchen floor and closed her eyes. Suddenly, she became overwhelmed by a vivid childhood memory of her father yelling at her after she had cleaned the kitchen.

Sitting on the kitchen floor crying, Angie began kicking the wall, and broke a bone in her left foot. Limping and in pain, she drove herself to the emergency room and told a nurse, Dot, "Just fix it so I can go to work Monday." Dot inquired and Angie disclosed what had happened, telling the nurse, "I don't know why I'm telling you all this." Dot then told Angie, "You need to promise me you'll see a therapist next week; here, I can give you a name." She talked Angie into promising to make an appointment, and when Angie said, "I'll go once; that's all," Dot told Angie that she should complete five appointments and "be honest about everything." Dot was the wife of a friend of mine and called to tell me that she had made the referral—not disclosing any other information, of course, except that Angie had committed to at least five appointments.

The intake meeting with Angie went smoothly, and she talked about her history without any hesitation. During the first part of the session after the intake, Angie reiterated what she had told Dot about her parents and made a statement that there was no hope for her, and nothing could help. The session included the following dialog:

Saul: Yes, this all sounds like a nightmare. Your parents' drinking and the way they treated you as a child were terrible. I can understand why you would believe that nothing will help;

that all you can do is work and not think about everything that happened. So, I need to ask: with all this in your past and everything that's been happening, how do you keep going every day?

Angie: I am barely making it. I told you; you now know more about my history probably than anyone. Nothing will change—it can't. Nothing will change. I will never be different. This is the way I will be for the rest of my life.

Saul: So, how do you manage to keep going—to get through each day?

Angie: I just have to keep my eye on the target and move on every single day. There's no hope for anything in my life to get much better. It's the way it is. I'll never be happy.

Saul: I know that's what you believe. I get it. It all sounds really challenging. So, what do you do to "keep your eye on the target and move on" every day?

Angie: I drink. I sleep. I go to work. I drink. That's how I do it. I hate my life. Nothing will be different. There is no hope for me.

Saul: You don't drink and sleep all day. You go to work.

Angie: I was told that I will never amount to anything. My dad was sure to tell me that I would never amount to anything. And my mom never loved me. She didn't defend me or say anything. I was the one who took care of them, and they hated me. Nothing will change in my life.

Saul: I believe that you think nothing will change. But you know, Angie, from where I sit, I don't think that I exactly agree with the idea that nothing will change; and we can talk more about that some other time. But I do have a question. I'm really curious: what do you do to get through each day? How do you even manage to get up in the morning?

Angie: I have to. I must go to work. It's not easy—I have to force myself to get up for work. I barely get up, get ready on time, and get out the door. It's an effort. It shouldn't be like this. I should be enjoying life like everyone else. I should be happy to get up in the morning and go to work. Life should be enjoyable.

Saul: I agree. Yes, you deserve better. Life should be enjoyable. I am wondering, how do you force yourself to get out of bed and get to work? Morning after morning, day after day. I am really impressed—even amazed, considering what you have been through. I think about the abuse you suffered; the alcoholic parents; the lack of nurturing; and all you've been through. How you manage to keep going, doing what you do, every day?

Angie: It's nothing—no big deal. I just force myself. I think of all the people who depend on me to deliver their packages. I have to get out of bed. I haven't missed a day's work for two years and I don't intend to. Even limping and hurt, I did my job last week. I have to—I don't really have much of a choice!

Saul: See, that's what I'm saying; that's what I'm wondering. How do you do it? How come things aren't worse? There are a lot of people who have difficulty getting to work on time—some who don't make it to work many days—and they haven't gone through anything like you have. It must say something about you.

Angie: You make it sound like some big thing. It's just what I have to do, so I just do it.

Saul: I see—it's because you are a person who makes up her mind and then just does it?

Angie: But only because I have to; not because I like it. I just do it.

Saul: Wow, Angie, that's great.

This exchange may sound somewhat discouraging, but it is promising and hopeful. Angie has revealed a key strength and perhaps a goal. She is a person who makes up her mind to do something and then just does it; and she believes that life should be enjoyable. Knowing those two things creates many possibilities for her in therapy. At the moment, she is consumed with her awful history and does not notice her personal power. From what I was able to see at the time, I hypothesized that she was looking for a way to "break out" of the doldrums and enjoy life. I made a mental note that her agenda might be that she wanted to be able to enjoy life. With that roadmap in mind, and knowing she was intelligent and insightful, I decided to use metaphor to assist her in thinking about the possibility that perhaps she could enjoy life.

I asked, "Angie, have you ever heard the story about the psychologist who put fleas in a jar?" She shook her head, indicating no. I began with the metaphor:

So, a psychologist put a bunch of fleas in a glass jar and put the lid on the jar. Of course, the fleas wanted to get out, so they jumped and jumped, over and over, all day and all night. But they kept hitting the inside of the lid and falling back to the bottom. He watched them. They jumped and jumped for three days. Then the psychologist took the lid off the jar. Do you know what happened?

Angie thought for a few seconds and said, "Hmmm—did they stop jumping?" I said, "No—they kept jumping. They wanted to get out. But they only jumped to where the lid used to be." Her eyes opened wide. I could see that she was reflecting on the story. Then she said, "That's like me, isn't it?" I replied, "One thing that's really different is that when you make up your mind to do something, you just do it, and you have free will." Angie smiled.

Angie began the intake meeting and her first therapy session as a visitor in relation to change, and as a complainant in relation to her "awful" history and the idea that she could enjoy life. As primarily a visitor at intake, I could only encourage her to return for the next appointment to explore "if meeting with me could be helpful." Angie's commitment to Dot that she would attend at least five sessions was probably helpful in bringing her back for another appointment. Angie had revealed previously hidden details of her history and, perhaps more importantly, some of her feelings about the abuse she had suffered. When Angie revealed that a piece of her agenda was about "enjoying life," she opened the door to eventually becoming a customer.

To help Angie continue on track for at least the few sessions that she had committed to attend, I decided on an observational task that would fit with her position as a complainant about her life and perhaps be compatible with her agenda. My goal was to offer Angie a task that would sharpen her perspective, identify some of her accomplishments to build hope, and perhaps motivate her more toward becoming a customer. I decided on a facsimile of Insoo Kim Berg's and Steve de Shazer's "standard first session task" that was first introduced at the Brief Family Therapy Center: "Between now and the next time we meet, I would like you to observe, so that you can describe to me next time, what is happening in your life that you like and want to continue to have happen." (de Shazer 1985, pp. 137-138)

Angie completed the task between sessions; and during the next meeting, she was able to list several things in her life that she liked and wanted to continue. In addition to her job, condominium, and good health, I was somewhat surprised to learn that she loved to read mystery novels; had a "green thumb and the best garden in town," and a season pass for the philharmonic orchestra; had a dog and two cats; and considered two coworkers good friends even though her primary contacts with them thus far had been to meet for lunch during the meal break at work.

I also learned that Angie had played the violin in middle school; and that her two friends at work, Jill and Tam, had invited her several times to a weekend activity but she had declined each time. I asked, "How come?" and she said, "I don't know." I responded with, "If you did know, what would you say?" Angie stared at me for a few seconds and then said, with some hesitancy, "I guess I thought they were just being polite." I responded with, "I see—so when they really mean it, when they want to have you join them, how will you know?" Angie turned her head to the side and then straightened up before responding, "You know, that's a good point. Next time they ask, I'll accept and find out if they really mean it."

I continued to ask Angie about her friends at work. My next questions were to learn what they talked about at lunch. Angie's first response was, "Not much; nothing important." I continued, "Angie, there must have been something that you can share with me." She answered, "I don't know." I again asked, "If you did know, what would you say?" Angie replied, "What? Again?" and laughed. Before I could respond, she said, "We've talked about a lot of things, but I didn't tell them about my family. I guess we do have some things in common. Maybe." Then she revealed several things that they had in common, including a love of music and novels. Each had read some books that the others had read, and they made book recommendations to each other. Rather than assigning her a task, I asked her, "What will happen next that will tell you that you're on track—that you've moved forward toward changing things in the direction you want them to go?" Angie said, "I'll do something outside of work with Jill and Tam, and I'll have a good time."

Angie returned a week later, and I asked her, "What's better?" She looked almost excited, which caught me off guard because she usually presented as serious and somewhat uncomfortable. She said:

> We went out to dinner together—Tam and Jill and me. It was fun. I can't remember ever laughing so much. Tam has a yard and she told me that she has a lot of work to do, so I offered to help her. And you wouldn't believe it, but Jill also played the violin in school, through high school so I'm sure she was much better than I could ever have been. Oh, and we're going to meet again this week for dinner.

I responded, "That sounds great!" Angie continued:

> Maybe I'll make them dinner at my place sometime. I used to be a pretty good cook. I learned to cook as a kid. Maybe I can get back into cooking for other people again without making a mess and flooding the place!

We both laughed. Then I responded, "Hey, you know—I can hear that maybe you're on your way to enjoying life? You were right when you said, 'Life should be enjoyable.' "

If there's any question about why I told Angie that she was right when she said, "Life should be enjoyable," I will own up to throwing success in her face. She had met her original agenda and at least temporarily filled the "sadness/loneliness hole in her heart." We still had other goals to define and issues to address, such as "drinking at night to fall asleep," "occasional flashbacks," and perhaps "issues with her family." There was no doubt in my mind that she would be able to tackle those concerns after she had seen her worth in the eyes of her peers. Her friends' acceptance provided a counterbalance to the "you will never amount to anything" message from her father.

In earlier chapters, I referenced Milton Erickson's idea that clients have all the strengths and resources they need to resolve their problems and succeed. In addition to agreeing with Erickson, I believe that when I can bring a client to imagine a time when the problem is not happening and to envision what change will look like, we can build hope, willingness, and new possibilities. I had collected information about Angie's strengths and resources, and then continued to reference them while searching for and processing exceptions to whatever problems she brought up. Following Angie's prompts, I could see that she was ready to address goal-setting questions. The next steps would include continuing to elicit solutions, and strategically having Angie identify ways to live into her solutions.

Angie did have everything she needed to break out of the chains from her past, but it required courage to take a risk and share her true self with two potentially close friends. Eventually, she disclosed her history of abuse and despair to Jill and Tam, learning that each of them had at least some similarities in their history. Angie appreciated that she was not the only "survivor," and came to understand that her childhood trauma did not define her. Her confidence and willingness to be more open accelerated, as did her healing. I continued to work with Angie over the following months as she continued to set concrete goals for herself through questions such as, "What else needs to happen for you to say that your life is enjoyable?" At each benchmark, the questions evolved into, "What will happen next for you to enjoy life even more? How will you be doing that?" Angie began to constructively confront and resolve things that bothered her. Encouraging her to build a vision for the future became important during the last few sessions before her discharge from treatment.

As it turned out, Jill had a six-year-old child, so both Tam and Angie acted as "assistant parents," wanting to help ensure that Jill's daughter had a wonderful childhood. About five years after Angie was discharged from therapy, I occasionally would see her in town. Eventually she was offered and accepted a management position somewhere and left the area.

Clients such as Angie are often treated as a diagnosis—perhaps in her circumstances as alcohol use disorder, depression, post-traumatic stress disorder, and social anxiety. Diagnosis is necessary for insurance payments, but it can get in the way of an authentic human connection and effective therapeutic alliance. Angie could have been attending therapy for years and still been drowning in problems to this day if a strict problem-focused intervention had been attempted. Viewing her as a competent person with everything she needed allowed for a strength-based, client-need-driven approach that revealed her strengths and supported her efforts to overcome a hurtful past. Specifically, what worked involved describing behaviors and issues rather than using labels; identifying and building on her strengths and resources; respecting her "position" and agenda; introducing metaphor and humor; and eliciting her ideas and solutions.

Solution process questions are set out in Appendix G.

Eleven-Year-Old Terry: Removing the Target on His Back

Advocating within the larger system can help a client overcome obstacles toward completing a significant goal. Therapists often miss opportunities to be helpful when clients are working toward substantive change but are unable to make headway because of a person or agency that has the power to interfere with or inadvertently sabotage their efforts. Therapists can be in the best place strategically to accomplish an intervention on a deserving client's behalf, but some define their role strictly and believe that it is not a clinician's role to advocate. My position has always been that a therapist who is genuinely committed to a vulnerable client's wellbeing should be willing to step outside the "45-minute hour" routine to make a difference.

One of my most memorable experiences in this arena involved an 11-year-old male foster child who was referred to me for counseling. Terry had been in foster care since age three and had been in several foster homes. His current foster parents said that they did not have the time to attend therapy sessions with him, and they complained to the Child Welfare case manager that they were having problems with him at home and in school because "he was not making enough of an effort." Hearing some of the details regarding his behavior at home, it sounded to me like Terry might have been seeking attention and approval, and likely had been feeling unwanted and unloved. The foster parents, in not so many words, indicated that they did not have any hope for him. It was clear that they did not want to be bothered with school problems, and the case manager was not going to intervene on Terry's behalf or challenge the foster parents' hopelessness. Their expectation of therapy was that I needed to find a way to improve Terry's behavior at home and convince him to do well in school.

I encouraged the foster parents to attend the first session after the intake, but they declined. It would have been helpful to have them available so Terry could see that they were partners in his efforts with me. During the next two meetings with Terry, I learned that over the years in various foster homes he had heard either directly or indirectly that he was a victim of an unfortunate past, with neglectful biological parents who did not love him. He showed sadness and appeared reluctant to accept that things could ever be much better. Terry's belief was reinforced from attending years of Child Welfare meetings, court hearings, and psychiatric evaluations—plus occasionally eavesdropping on phone conversations or discussions in his foster homes. When Terry spoke of hopelessness, I noted that he referenced what others had said; but he was not self-deprecating, and in my presence never indicated feeling defective or unworthy.

I asked Terry, "How come things aren't worse, with all you've been through? How come you are so well-spoken, smart, and personable?" His answer surprised me. "If I tell you, will you keep quiet about it? I must know that. Promise me." I explained to him again the protections and limits of confidentiality from the intake session, and Terry said:

> That's what I thought; I figured you could keep quiet about my private stuff. Right? Well, I think that they are not talking about me; they're talking about their opinion or maybe what would happen to other people. I know that, and I've learned to keep things to myself when I know too much. You have to be careful around these people because they think everything means a symptom and I need help. Or they accuse me of trying to manipulate. Words are useless because you can't prove anything to them with words. Telling them doesn't prove anything, no matter what I try to tell them. I've stopped trying to tell them. The reason things are not worse is because I can take care of myself and understand how this all works.

I complimented Terry on how strong, smart, and insightful he was; and I promised him that I would be sure to listen and understand without judging or stereotyping him. "You have so many attributes and strengths, in spite of everything," I told him. He said, " 'Stereotyping'—that's the word. That's what people do to me. Not you; other people." I made a clear, verbal agreement with Terry that things would be different with me, and it would be safe for him to say what was on his mind. I empathized how difficult it must be to go through "all this muck," and then stated that it was a good thing he was so strong and smart. "Terry," I asked, "what needs to happen for you to make a clear statement without words to show that you are strong and smart?" He thought for a few seconds and then said, "I can do better in school. Maybe that will matter; maybe then they'll know that I'm okay and not all messed up."

I nodded and told Terry:

> It must be hard when people have so much power over you but I'm confident you are up to the task. I'll support whatever you need in order to make the statement you want to make to them or anyone else. Things

will be different, very different now that you are taking charge of your life and future.

For the next few weeks, I saw Terry open up to me and glow with pride when I gave him approval. It was clear that he had rarely been complimented. I encouraged him to continue his good efforts. Terry became willing to take appropriate risks around getting closer to people while at the same time acknowledging how the circumstances of his past were affecting his life now. He was very intelligent—beyond his years—and understood the cause and effect of his history and current situation. He was motivated to overcome the limitations that others had imposed on him.

Terry was making good progress in therapy and initiated a discussion of how he had stood up to some of the painful things in his life. His expression changed to a confident tone, and he began to believe that things could get better because he could make them better. He was not hesitant to try "experiments" to check out if he could improve relationships with other adults through changes to his behavior and temperament. Terry's efforts were paying off in almost every setting: Boys and Girls Club, Little League, Youth Basketball, Latchkey, and even his foster home. But in school, his efforts were not bearing fruit, and he was getting frustrated. We talked about his counselor and teacher; from what I could tell, Terry was doing his part by working harder and participating, but they were not responding fully to his positive changes. He asked if I could help him by telling them that he was trying to be a better student and person. I thought that was a magnificent idea; and I told him that if I had his permission to tell them he was in therapy with me, I would meet with them.

There was some "red tape" involved because the state had legal and physical custody of Terry, but I was able to get the Department of Child and Family Services (DCFS) to sign a consent form so I could talk to the school about Terry and get information from them. I knew better than to ask DCFS for anything more specific than permission to coordinate my efforts with the school. Whenever a child in the state's custody was a client, I would donate my time and intervene if advocacy would help. My experience informed me that I needed to carefully word all requests. I wrote on the consent form that I needed to "disclose details regarding Terry's behavior and the progress I had noticed in response to therapy and collect information on his school behaviors and progress." Public agencies can be territorial or try to second-guess the work of professionals. My actual plan involved some strategies that I was not confident they would understand—at least not initially.

I waited until Monday morning and visited first with the school counselor. Explaining who I was and providing him with the consent forms, I engaged the counselor in a conversation about Terry. He confirmed my suspicions: there was no acknowledgment of the improved efforts and progress that I knew Terry had made. I could have shown the counselor copies of homework and in-class essays that I had collected, but instead I said:

> I need a favor so that I can help Terry. He's been attending therapy with me and recently has had some impressive breakthroughs. His courage to face his past and deal with his hurts is remarkable. He is making a big effort to turn things around; but he's afraid that you and his teacher won't even notice—after all, there are so many students, and you are so busy with important things. I told Terry that you would want to help, but he is afraid his efforts won't matter so he gave me permission to talk to you. It would help if you could notice his efforts and improvements, and prepare a list every week that I could pick up on Friday afternoon. Then I will share the list with Terry during our weekly sessions to show him that you do notice. I believe that will help him to have confidence that hard work can make a difference in school. Could you do that for Terry and me?

Terry's counselor agreed wholeheartedly with my plan, so I asked him if I could speak to Terry's teacher to ask if she would do the same. He arranged for me to see Terry's teacher and I explained things to her in the same way. She agreed to notice Terry's efforts and improvements every week, and to get a list to his counselor by noon every Friday so I could pick up the lists at the same time. They both appeared appropriately concerned about Terry's situation and willing to help. In essence, I was assigning a "notice" task to the school in a similar way that I would assign it to a "complainant" in a family.

Of course, asking his counselor and teacher to notice Terry's efforts and improvement worked to help them pay attention to anything even remotely positive. As their attitude toward Terry improved, Terry's attitude toward them and school also improved. When I read their comments to Terry each week, and complimented him on what they had noticed, he became more and more motivated to succeed in school. I could see the emotion in his teary eyes as I read to him the positive comments from the counselor and teacher.

Terry's drive was fueled by their acknowledgments plus their implied expectation that he was becoming a top student who would be successful. In meeting with me, Terry shared a newfound love for school, and admiration for his teacher and counselor. I could hear from Terry's disclosures that both the counselor and teacher were making additional time for him and complimenting his work. He just missed straight As in the next grading period; but in his first semester in seventh grade, he achieved straight As. Intervention with his school turned into a life changer for him!

The foster parents informed the case manager that Terry's behavior and attitude had significantly improved. I was invited to a team meeting; and because the school personnel were unable to attend, I was asked to report on Terry's achievements in school. I also discussed his progress in therapy and the courage he had displayed in confronting a difficult history and an uncertain future. The written report I submitted outlined his progress and provided a very positive prognosis.

When the foster parents were asked, they discussed Terry's improvements in attitude and behavior in their home. The case manager complimented the foster parents on their "excellent work to turn Terry around" without openly giving Terry credit. Near the end of the meeting, I asked to make a statement. I addressed my words to Terry:

> Terry, you are now 12 years old, and you have accomplished the growth in one year that might take most people a lifetime to achieve. You have shown great maturity for your years and the courage of a lion! I have witnessed your hard work. I have witnessed the completion of your worthy goals. You have kept every promise that you made to me. Nobody can deny your determination and resilience. People are noticing your successes. You have a bright future ahead. I am proud and honored to have gotten to know you!

References

De Jong, P. and Berg, I. K. (2013). *Interviewing for Solutions*. 4th Ed. Belmont, CA: Brooks/Cole.

de Shazer, S. (1985). *Keys to Solution in Brief Therapy*. New York: Norton.

8 Children of Juvenile Justice and Child Welfare

Structural Family Dynamics

Structural family assessments can help us to understand how the parental hierarchy and child subsystem influence the balance and functioning of the family. "Dysfunction" can be defined as the product of an imbalance in the family structure. The "unnatural" roles that family members—primarily children—are forced to take in order to balance and "save the family system" have a lifelong influence on the child. The more common roles are family scapegoat, hero, mascot, or lost child (Woititz 1983).

It is preferable to use the term "functional" rather than "healthy" to characterize a family that is safe and nurturing, and that meets the needs of its members. Functional families can have a single parent; have two parents of any gender and marital status; or be non-traditional in terms of caretakers. There is no single design to a "functional" family. Families of any parental configuration can also be dysfunctional. Regardless, when children experience neglect, abuse, or any form of emotional or physical abandonment—especially from a caretaker—they are profoundly affected. Conversely, families that have at least one nurturing parent in the parental hierarchy, providing protection, nurturing, and love to children in the child subsystem, can offer sound potential for appropriate development throughout the stages of childhood.

One possible variable to keep in mind is that, depending on a child's age and life experiences, adoption can complicate family dynamics and child-parent issues. Adoptive children may be internalizing and reacting to the dynamics of both their adoptive and biological family. Children with severe trauma prior to adoption, and those diagnosed with reactive attachment disorder, often will face additional challenges regardless of the structure and dynamics of the adoptive family, or how well meaning and caring the adoptive parents might be. Their issues will likely require specific, specialized intervention.

To illustrate structural family dynamics, we will look at a traditional two-parent family. It is important to understand that, whether a family

DOI: 10.4324/9781003397380-8

is traditional or non-traditional—such as single parent, same-sex parents, step-parents, or adoptive parents—it is the relationships of adults to adults, adults to children, children to adults, and children to children that primarily determine function or dysfunction, and ultimately the roles children might be susceptible to acquire. The composition of the family matters less than the family dynamics and experiences that will affect the children emotionally.

The structural view of a functional traditional family might be illustrated as follows:

Father		Mother	
Child	Child	Child	Child

The line represents a functional boundary between the parental hierarchy and the child subsystem. The father (F) and mother (M) are above the boundary line, and the children (C) are below the boundary line in the child subsystem. Parents are the caretakers, and the children can function as children.

Hypothetically, let's say one of the parents—in this example, the father—is addicted to substances and is emotionally unavailable. Consequently, he is disengaging emotionally from the family; and we will assume for this illustration that he requires care, protection, and "rescuing" from the other parent. Mother must be the primary parent for the children and at the same time a "parent-enabler" to the father, taking on many if not all the adult family responsibilities. Essentially, the father is now part of the child subsystem:

	Mother		
Father	Child	Child	Child	Child

When a system is out of balance, children take on new roles in an effort to help—even save—their family. In this example, two things are likely to happen next.

One of the children may send a "cry for help" by taking on the family's emotional burden. This child will "act out" in order to bring attention to the family, while providing cover for the addicted, dysfunctional parent by looking like the "problem." This child might be clinically described as overly sensitive, attention seeking, or self-sacrificing; but society will likely focus on the troubled behavior and characterize the child as "delinquent." During adolescence, this is the child who might become addicted to substances and act promiscuously. Some social systems might conclude that the problem is this child, not the family, and attempt to "fix" the child's behavior by focusing services on the child. The role played by this child is the family "scapegoat."

The family structure would thus look like this:

Mother				
Father	Child	Child	Child	Ch. Scapegoat

In this illustration, mother is the lone parent in the parental hierarchy and is overwhelmed. One of the other children may then attempt to be her helper and move into the parental hierarchy. This child is the responsible or "perfect" child: succeeding in school, behaving well, and acting as a surrogate parent to help raise the children and take on family responsibilities usually reserved for a parent. This child also provides cover for the dysfunctional parent and family by appearing strong and together. Neighbors and school personnel might conclude, "How can there be anything wrong with this family—look how well that child is doing?" The "hero" attempts to give the family "self-worth," ensuring that adult responsibilities are met. If Child Welfare or Mental Health becomes involved, they might notice this child's caretaker responsibilities and label them "parentified." More likely, outsiders will see this child as "perfect," "mature," and "mommy's little helper." The role this child plays is the "hero."

The family structure would then look like this:

Mother	Ch. Hero		
Father	Child	Child	Ch. Scapegoat

Depending on the needs, characteristics, and dynamics of the family, either the scapegoat or the hero will appear first—although sometimes those roles emerge concurrently.

Families experiencing the stress of a parent overwhelmed and grieving, a second parent who is needy with addictive behaviors, and children in protective roles scrambling to help usually lack humor and fun. A third child may attempt to fill that void by adding fun, entertainment, and even hope by being a star athlete, or a little ballerina, or a stage entertainer, or a comedian. That child provides distraction from problems, while at the same time providing cover to the family and trying to build the illusion of wellbeing. Family members will often come together at sporting or theater events and appear to be getting along and functioning well. The role this placating child plays is "mascot."

The family structure would then look like this:

Mother	Ch. Hero		
Father	Child	Ch. Mascot	Ch. Scapegoat

Families with a structural imbalance at some point will become overwhelmed. Taking on any additional responsibilities would be too formidable. Children usually possess keen sensitivities and are the first to be emotionally impacted by dynamics that threaten their family. Once again, it will be a child who comes to the rescue. One of the children will withdraw and fade into the background, not make any "waves," and seek to become as invisible as possible in school, home, and socially. This is the "invisible" child, who is quiet and hardly noticed, does not bring attention to themselves, and provides relief to everyone in the family through the solitude of not requiring attention. Sometimes referred to as quiet, invisible, or perfect, this child adopts the role of the "lost child."

Mother	Ch. Hero		
Father	Ch. Lost Child	Ch. Mascot	Ch. Scapegoat

Children adopt roles to balance the family system and allow it to function, but at their own peril. In order to address the needs of the family, children can play multiple roles and even share or switch roles—certainly when there are fewer than four children, or when one of the children temporarily leaves home or ages out and lives independently. As unlikely as it may sound, a child can even alternate between the role of scapegoat and hero. It can be challenging for a clinician to assess history or current family circumstances when a child plays more than one role concurrently or when children switch roles.

Children do not automatically shed their childhood roles when they become adults. The same children, now grown up as adult children of alcoholic parents (ACOAs) or parents with other compulsive behaviors, maintain the essence of the roles that dominated their feelings, behaviors, self-concept, self-worth, and choices in childhood. Often overlooked are children of workaholic parents, who can experience a similar outcome because workaholism—as with any addiction or compulsion—manifests as emotionally and/or physically dysfunctional parenting. In Chapter 9, we discuss in detail how childhood roles can spill over into adulthood and have a profound effect on the lives of ACOAs.

Treatment Needs to Address the Whole Family

Creative clinicians such as Sal Minuchin, M.D. (1984) pioneered an understanding of the structural family system, and how behaviors and family functioning are negatively impacted when the parental hierarchy and child subsystem are out of alignment. Dr. Minuchin's (1974) original work and teachings in this area are unparalleled. Throughout his life, the work he did with families was groundbreaking. I was personally inspired by his commitment to minorities and families living in poverty. Dr. Minuchin was readily available to young clinicians and shared his findings and methods in presentations and workshops.

One of the interventions that he shared at a workshop had a significant impact on me. In the 1990s, he was asked to assess children who had been in mental health facilities in New York for considerable periods of time. The boy in a video (let's call him Timmy) was about ten years old and had been confined in the hospital for two years. Dr. Minuchin's interaction with the boy could hardly be called an interview because Timmy was so medicated that he appeared zombie-like, and his speech was slow and flat. Timmy could not answer the question, "Why are you here?" He was genuinely too confused and dazed to carry on a conversation. It was emotionally wrenching to watch.

Dr. Minuchin then interviewed the hospital psychiatrist responsible for Timmy's care and confirmed that Timmy was not and had not been a danger to himself or others. He referenced hyperactivity and impulsivity as a reason for hospitalization. Dr. Minuchin then asked about Timmy's treatment plan and care; and the psychiatrist answered that Timmy was still not showing much improvement despite trials with several medications, and most recently a combination of psychotropic medications. He boasted about "titrating" different medications in combination to attempt to find the right mixture for behavioral control and reduction of symptoms. The psychiatrist had a flat affect and did not display what I would have called appropriate compassion or concern. This was also emotionally difficult for me to observe.

Timmy's mother was then interviewed, and talked about how sad she was that her son was hospitalized and not living with her. Dr. Minuchin asked, "Why is Timmy here? What is the reason?" and Timmy's mother answered, "Because I could not control him." Dr. Minuchin then said to her, "Let me see if I understand. Timmy has been here for two years. He is here because you cannot control him. Is that correct?" Timmy's mother acknowledged that Dr. Minuchin understood correctly. Dr. Minuchin then said, "Your son is here because you, his mother, cannot control him. How come you are not here?" The mother did not know how to respond; but in addition to being flustered, I had the impression that she was reflecting on the question. The significance of the question was impactful. Dr. Minuchin's writings and intervention ideas will always be an influence on my thinking about children and families.

One tendency in children who are separated from their family is that they invariably want to be returned to their parents. Rarely does the abuse, neglect, rejection, or dysfunction matter. Children usually want their family back. We see this tendency in Child Welfare, Juvenile Justice, and Mental Health. Professionals in public agencies that protect children or society may correctly assess that the risk is too high to allow reunification. But then again, at 18 or whatever the age of majority is, there is a good chance that the child will return home regardless of what the "system" does. If we listen to the kids, they are saying that we need to address and improve the functioning of their families because all the "rescuing" will likely not keep them from returning home.

When I worked at Youth Parole, we were given a directive that the child was our primary client/ward, so requiring the family's presence in counseling was not encouraged. The structure of the juvenile justice system in general focused on the youth and the behavior of the youth outside the context of the family. If it was determined that the juvenile was not complying with the probation or parole agreement—perhaps involving school truancy, drug and alcohol abuse, incorrigibility at home, and runaway or theft offenses—they were then sent away to a treatment facility to be confined and receive rehabilitation services.

Testing, counseling, and peer support services with activities were provided at the youth correctional facility. There was a fully accredited high school on the campus, and the youth were required to attend classes taught by high-school teachers. Most of them did very well in school, received compliments on their behavior, participated in constructive activities, and got along with peers. When they returned home, there was a strong expectation that lasting behavioral changes had occurred. Invariably, following a short "honeymoon period," many of the youth regressed to their old behaviors. A family system's homeostasis—its need for restorative balance—is powerful. The changes that the youth had made were temporary because they were subordinate to the needs and dynamics of the family system. Unchanged family dynamics resulted in the children being thrust into the familiar, pre-treatment role.

These and other real-world observations, coupled with the ideas, concepts, and research by the founders of family systems therapy, drove my practice standards for children who were presented as "identified patients" by their families. I would not allow parents to bring their child to therapy and leave. My condition, for the sake of the child and family, was that the parents—and, when appropriate, the other children in the family—had to attend therapy together. Some of the strategies that have been successful in working with families facing extraordinary challenges are discussed in later chapters, and in the story of Ashley's family below.

Barely a Teen

A young teen and her family were referred to me for therapy. Ashley had just turned 15 and had been on juvenile probation for two years. At 13 years old, as an eighth grader, she had been arrested as a suspect in a teenage burglary ring. Shortly after her arrest, an investigation showed that Ashley had not been involved directly in the home burglaries, but had accepted stolen property from her friends who had been "adjudicated delinquent" for commiting several burglaries. Ashley admitted to the court that recently she had a few beers "for the first time" because she did not want to seem "chicken" to her friends. She denied using drugs, although her probation officer believed that she smoked pot with the friends who had been committing burglaries.

Ashley's parents had cooperated with the police and Juvenile Probation, and 13-year-old Ashley complied with a referral for individual counseling as part of the original probation agreement. A young female alcohol and drug counselor, Megan, was thought to be the best choice for her. Ashley had attended individual counseling weekly for almost a year when she was discharged by the counselor, who noted that Ashley was not really invested in counseling. Probation had asked the counselor to address with Ashley her possible use of pot and her continued contact with the friends who had participated in the burglaries. Three males and four females— teens between one and two years older than Ashley—were identified by the Juvenile Probation officer as the "problems." Ashley had been jeopardizing her probation by maintaining contact with the older teens on probation.

Ashley was then referred to another clinician: a psychologist who was well established in the community, and who was often selected by Juvenile Probation to evaluate teens who had been arrested. The psychologist did some testing and after three months determined that Ashley was not going to be cooperative in therapy. Her report stated that Ashley had expressed some disappointment in herself, but had a loyalty bond to her friends and would not give them up or implicate them in any way. She also noted that Ashley did not agree with the idea that she had done anything wrong by accepting stolen items, but at the same time acknowledged that burglary is wrong. In her report, the psychologist characterized Ashley as defiant, naïve, selfish, uncooperative, and immature. Her diagnoses included oppositional defiant with a "ruleout" for borderline personality disorder, which I found to be inappropriate.

Ashley had been a C and D student during the two years since her arrest; but in sixth and seventh grade she had been a straight "A" student and her teachers considered her very intelligent and motivated. She had just turned 15 years old and, according to her parents, was more evasive and defiant than ever, with an attitude that she could do whatever she wanted. One night, Ashley was caught by her parents after sneaking out of her house. Her parents waited through the night and watched as she climbed back into her room through the window the next morning. They confronted her and there was a fierce argument. Ashley superficially scraped her arms with a knife later that day and was booked into Juvenile Detention for protective custody.

Ashley's mother had been experiencing feelings of dispair, difficulty sleeping, and loss of appetite, which she attributed to worrying about Ashley. She had been attending individual therapy for more than four months. Ashley's mother was making progress and some of her symptoms were no longer as intense. She expressed love for Ashley and a willingness to make whatever constructive changes might be necessary; but she made it clear that she and her husband had tried but were at a loss to find a way to improve Ashley's behavior. Mom's therapist gave them my name and suggested they call me, cautioning that I would be asking to see the whole family together. Ashley's mom promised to call me, but expressed some concern about her husband being able to attend all therapy sessions because he worked long hours and often did not get home until late.

When Ashley's parents called and explained the situation, I agreed to work with Ashley on three conditions: that I received a copy of the files from Ashley's previous therapists; that the parents would refer to our meetings as "family therapy," rather than therapy for Ashley; and that all of them would attend every appointment together unless we agreed on some other arrangement. I also talked with them about the informed consent paperwork that would need to be signed by each family member, and suggested that they inform Ashley's probation officer as soon as they start counseling with me.

When the family came in for their first appointment, there was a surprise. Four people showed up. Ashley had a brother, Doug, eight years old. There was no reference to him in the intake papers from the previous therapists, and no reference to him in the probation and court documents the family had given to me. Neither parent had mentioned him during our telephone exchange. I had to guess that he was truly the classic "lost child." During family therapy sessions, Ashley sat next to him and checked in on him often, wanting to make sure he was doing okay and asking him if he understood what was being said or if he had any questions. Ashley's parents barely looked at him, and did not discuss anything about him or with him during our exchanges.

Ashley looked much younger than her years. I would have guessed her age at about 12 based on her physical appearance, but she was very intelligent and very sophisticated for her age. She opened the first session during introductions by saying, "Don't ask me to give up my friends; you can't make me give them up. Don't tell me what I can't do." Her parents tried to defend me by saying, "Ashley, Saul has a job to do." Mom then tried to reassure me by saying, "Please be patient with her; my therapist told me that being in high school has just enboldened her."

I got to see two sides of Ashley: the teen whose body language was rigid and words were impatient and defiant, not wanting to engage with me and clearly not wanting to be in my office with her parents; and a nurturing big sister with sensitive, compassionate feelings for her kid brother, checking in on him and being protective. Ashley was not happy to meet me but I could discern that she was curious about my methods and listened intently.

Ashley's parents expressed their concern for Ashley and described the problem as: "We no longer can control Ashley and she is ruining her life; if she would stop sneaking around and seeing her delinquent friends, that would help." Doug described the problem as: "My parents can't control Ashley, and Ashley is a good person who loves me and has friends." Ashley described the problem as: "Everybody wants me to give up my friends and they are my friends; they are not bad people and my probation officer and parents need to get over it." Ashley had already stated that she was willing to go to the mat and not give up her friends; so it was clear that regardless of whose "agenda" that was, it would only provoke defiance in Ashley if I brought it up directly.

The family was asked the question, "What needs to happen for you to say that the problem that brought you here is resolved and you don't need to come here anymore?" Ashley's parents answered: "Ashley would again be doing well in school, be responsible, and not be sneaking around to see those friends." Doug said, "Ashley would be happy and my parents would be happy. She is my hero." Ashley said, "Everyone would get off my case—just leave me alone—and I would really be a hero to Doug."

The second meeting got off to a rocky start. Ashley was angry and sat down defiantly. She folded her arms and contorted her facial muscles to show the intensity of her anger. She glared at me. "What's up?" I asked. "You work for the court, don't you?" she said. I told her "no" and asked what gave her that impression. "My probation officer told me that I had to cooperate with you. You promised me that being here wouldn't be about my probation." It took much of that session just to clear things up; but I decided that I liked Ashley's spirit, and loved that she was so open about her concerns. I complimented her more than once for being honest with me. I could see her attitude soften and she even smiled a couple of times when I brought humor into the family discussions. I ended the session by saying, "Ashley, please be patient with me. I'm trying to find out what you want so that I can be helpful. I want things to work out well for you on your terms." She smiled and nodded, then looked at her parents for their reaction. At that point, I knew that we would have a successful outcome.

Session three was groundbreaking. After that meeting I wrote in my progress notes:

> Parents were more calm and willing to listen without trying to inter-ject concerns. Ashley is concerned about her little brother Doug, eight years old, who looks up to her. Ashley is afraid that her brother will be susceptible to bad influences when he is her age, and get into "real trouble." She characterized him as "too innocent to understand." Doug told Ashley that she is his hero, and she again made it clear that she wants to be a hero for him and make a difference.

I believed that I had found Ashley's "agenda" and would be able to work with her in a more effective way. Her "agenda" was to be a "hero" to Doug, and I needed to learn from Ashley the details of what that entailed and how I could be helpful. But before I could process direct questions about her agenda, it would be important to change things up a little. When families have had a history of intense disagreements and conflicts, I have looked to non-verbal strategies to help communicate information that might otherwise be difficult for them to process and accept. One method, for example, could be family sculpting, which involves family members moving and positioning one another as if making a sculpture of their family. But for this family, I was considering an alternative to sculpting because I wanted an intervention that would take less time and immedi-ately be compatible with addressing Ashley's agenda.

Beginning with the fourth session, I decided to use a strategy that I had learned from structural family therapist Maurizio Andolfi, M.D. (1979). In therapy, he often arranged seating and positioned a family into the structure that reflected their actual family dynamics. Dr. Andolfi was also known to "honor the voices of children in therapy," believing that they were the means to unlocking the family issues and igniting positive change. I began with the parental dyad by moving mom and dad's chairs to the edges of the room, next to one another. In the center of the room, I placed Ashley's chair directly across from and facing mine, and moved Doug behind me just off to the side so that he would be only in Ashley's view, blocked from the parent's line of sight and behind me. This arrangement mirrored exactly the presenting family structure, with the parents close together looking at Ashley, and not seeing Doug. Only Ashley could see and notice Doug.

I proceeded to process Ashley's agenda while her parents observed. As I got into a dialog with Ashley and she began to disclose, one or both of her parents would interrupt and either add to her disclosure or try to correct her perceptions. From my perspective, the parents were well-meaning but were interrupting Ashley's processing during the session. It was likely that they had been unwittingly interrupting Ashley's processes throughout adolescence; and perhaps her defiance had been about individuating and bringing attention to her family. So, out of necessity, I implemented talking rules. The basic rule was that Ashley and I were going to have a one-to-one talk, and her parents were to notice Ashley's ideas and wisdom without responding. Doug was asked to watch his sister and notice how loving a person she was—notably how much she cared about him.

I began with a review of Ashley's idea that she needed to be a hero to her brother and then scaled by asking, "On a 'hero' scale of 0-10, with 0 being not at all a hero and 10 being the hero you need to be to Doug, where are you today?" Ashley said, "I'm a 2." I then "anchored" the number by asking her, "So what's happening that makes you a 2?" Ashley stated:

> I love my brother and I try to protect him. I'm there for him and make sure he is taken care of and is safe. I pay attention to what is going on with him in his life and he knows I care. I make sure he doesn't do anything dangerous.

Then I processed and explored her answers by asking for specific examples of how she did those things. I followed up incrementally through number 5, starting with, "When you are a 3—a 'hero' up one more digit—what will be different? What will be happening to make you a 3?"

Ashley had a well-imagined picture of Doug's life ahead, likely modeled after some of her struggles growing up. When she was processing what a 5 was, she said:

> As Doug gets older, things will be harder for him. I know because they were for me. I guess unless I am a good role model, I can't really be his hero. I didn't have anyone for me. Maybe I've already screwed this up. Maybe he'll do the same things I did or worse. I don't know.

Then we ran out of time.

The fifth session began with the family entering quietly and proceeding to their pre-assigned seats. I checked in with everyone, and asked the parents if they had anything they would like to say. Dad began by offering to reconsider the way things were in the home and with their relationship toward their children. Mom affirmed what dad had said as she moved her chair so she could look at both Doug and Ashley. Then, mom said that things would be different, and Ashley would be respected. She looked at me, then Ashley, and told her that they would listen to her ideas. She added, "Doug is our son, and we love him. I guess that we were so focused on, worried about Ashley that we've sort of neglected him. It won't happen again. We are a family."

Doug talked about how nice his parents had been, and told me about a family day at the movies and an evening in an arcade during the previous week. Ashley smiled warmly and then asked me, "What happens now?" I said, "It's up to you, Ashley. You've taken us a long way, through a lot of issues that seem to be resolved now. It's up to you where we go next. Your parents are listening. They hear you."

Ashley looked at her parents and talked about how different today felt to her compared with the previous months and years. She acknowledged that things had been difficult for everyone and said that she did not know why "it had to happen like this." Then she turned to Doug and said, "Doug, I'm going to change so you can have a better life. It's my choice. I want this. I'll be there for you. Always." Then she looked me firmly in the eyes and said:

> Not for my probation officer and not for anyone but Doug, I will give up those friends—the ones I got into trouble with. And I won't be a friend to anyone who gets into trouble. I hope it's not too late.

Doug smiled. Her mom cried. Her dad put his arm around his wife. I nodded with acknowledgment and turned to Doug, telling him, "Your sister must really love you."

We had two more meetings together. The next session was to reaffirm the family's positive direction through compliments and a review of their strengths and resilience. The last session afforded me the opportunity to hear the family's joy and optimism. I could see in their interaction the structural correction they had made. The family had naturally repositioned their chairs so that all of them were in view of each other. There was a functional balance with the parental hierarchy and child subsystem. Mom and dad both addressed Doug and his concerns during our discussions. Ashley was released from probation six months later and kept her word to Doug and her parents. She put her life back on track and went off to college after graduating from high school.

When I had reviewed the notes of Ashley's previous therapists, what came to mind was a picture of a rowboat. Ashley had one of the oars, and the therapists had the other oar. Ashley was rowing clockwise on one side of the boat, and the therapists were rowing counterclockwise on the other side, causing the boat to go in circles. Working toward behavioral change requires all parties to row in the same direction. Addressing the reason for referral is not necessarily what will turn the corner. Learning what the client is invested in and invested in doing, what is meaningful to the client, and what will matter or make a difference is often more important than the actual reason for the referral.

Ashley's parents were focused on "fixing" Ashley; but in doing so, they had been neglecting Doug. Ashley had a "higher purpose," which was to correct her family structure and bring attention to Doug. She had taken whatever position and role was needed in an attempt to correct her family. To paraphrase a well-known comment that I've heard from Sal Minuchin (1984) when he described family members struggling to resolve a problem: *everyone was a good person, trying to do the right thing*. Working with the whole family together, addressing their structural issues, tending to the family's functioning, listening to Ashley's and the family's agendas, and allowing the family to correct itself are what made the therapy work.

References

Andolfi, M., (1979). *Family Therapy: An Interactive Approach*. New York: Plenum Press.

Minuchin, S. (1984). *Family Kaleidoscope*. Cambridge, MA: Harvard University Press.

Woititz, J. G. (1983). *Adult Children of Alcoholics*. Deerfield Beach, FL: Health Communications Inc.

9 Lacy and Grandma's Turkey
Family System Concepts

An understanding of family systems concepts and systems dynamics is invaluable when working with families, couples, and children. It is likewise critical to apply family systems thinking when working with clients in Child Welfare, Juvenile Justice, and any other programs that address family issues. Often, these agencies focus their interventions on the individual rather than the family. Rules and roles we internalize and function by; how we see ourselves in relation to others; our acceptance of or reluctance to change; openness and communication preferences; and our own parenting styles and family dynamics are strongly influenced by our family of origin. It is essential for clinicians to let the client or family teach us about their hierarchy, rules, and standards before we collaboratively develop a treatment plan. Typically, my workshop handouts for "family systems considerations" include the following:

- We all function in several contexts that influence us in many ways.
- How we function in each environment is impacted by all others, how we see our roles, and the rules of life that we have learned
- All systems tend toward homeostasis—the pull to stay the same and resist change.
- Although systems may tend to be either open or closed in general, systems can be open or closed around specific issues.
- Look at the whole to understand.
- If you change one part, other parts will change (commonly after trying to force change back to the outdated but familiar way).
- The whole is greater than the sum of the parts (the stuff between people).
- Systems have hierarchies, boundaries, rules, and roles.
- Systems are constantly challenged from the inside and outside.
- Systems are adaptive.

DOI: 10.4324/9781003397380-9

Communication Styles and Behaviors

How we communicate is often a combination of our family teachings, geographical styles, religious teachings, cultural norms, and social mores. I like to break it down simply: communication styles include emotive, reflective, supportive, and directive. Although most people have one dominant communication style, some use two or more styles under varying circumstances. There is no "right or wrong" communication style, although misunderstandings and conflicts can manifest between persons when styles are incompatible. Therapists need to assess and work compatibly with a client's communication style.

Non-verbal communication behaviors are also learned in the family and are an important part of family culture. Eye contact, social distancing, and touching are examples of communication behaviors. The meaning of communication behaviors can vary among cultures. For example, eye contact can be considered disrespectful in certain cultures; whereas a lack of eye contact can be considered disingenuous in others. Words and phrases can also have very different meanings in different cultures or even different parts of the country. Families and cultures tend to differ in the type and amount of information communicated directly through words or implicitly through non-verbal cues.

Most but not all of us in the United States and Europe are "low-context" communicators: we say somewhat directly, with words, what we mean. A low-context communicator might say: "Be sure to get to work on time if you want to get ahead"; or, "It's better to have a sure thing than to risk ending up with nothing." Low-context communicators are known for brevity and directness with words.

High-context communicators use metaphor or storytelling to make their point. They communicate indirectly, and often use more words to make a point than low-context communicators. Some of their "messages" can sound cryptic and contain 100 words or more. The choice of metaphor is likely based on their environment: a high-context communicator who lives in a community that farms or hunts will probably use the outdoor environment in their metaphors. For example, they might say: "The early bird catches the worm"; or "A bird in the hand is better than two in the bush." The messages from both a low-context communicator and a high-context communicator may attempt to say the same thing, but they will differ in style.

High-context communicators might think that a low-context communicator is rude because the direct message might sound confrontational and abrupt within their verbal culture. Low-context communicators might think that a high-context communicator is avoidant and trying to be evasive or "cute" rather than facing up to the situation. When a client and therapist use different styles, there is great potential for misunderstanding.

Lacy and the Story of Grandma's Turkey

The 1970s and 1980s were a time of rising divorce rates, and it was generally accepted that personal therapy would help recently separated and divorced persons to resolve grief and adjust to new challenges. In my private practice, I facilitated two process groups for divorcing clients in which we processed feelings, normalized issues, and worked toward resolution. Family of origin and generational issues were sometimes discussed by group members, with questions around "why" certain behaviors and attitudes seemed to surface and fester in intimate relationships. Lacy was especially interested in how dysfunctional behavior patterns developed and why "letting go" seemed so challenging. Working with her taught me about high-context communication styles, and a practical way to understand how family system behaviors and traditions can be dysfunctional and outdated yet continue to repeat in future generations.

Lacy grew up in Appalachia. She was a high-context communicator, and I was sometimes challenged—as were her group members—to understand the totality of her communications. There were underlying messages and symbolism, and Lacy seemed to cherish the questions that her group members would ask her. Some of her metaphors were unfamiliar or seemed out of context; but once clarified, they made a point. Sometimes I had to focus and think "outside the box" to understand what she was trying to say—or actually, what she was trying to teach.

Lacy seemed to enjoy the role of teacher or "guru." Unsurprisingly, she was the first child in her family to complete high school and had even earned an AA degree from a community college. Her role, as the brightest child in her family, was to be the hero and "teacher" for her siblings and parents. There was a mystical air to Lacy's metaphors and stories, and we never knew if they were true or just made up—although she claimed everything was true. She was smart and interesting; yet confounding at times.

Thanksgiving approached and several of the group members did not have family in the area. Lacy informed the group that she had a tradition of inviting friends to her house for Thanksgiving, but only on the condition that she did all of the cooking, and they brought a salad and dessert. Recently divorced, Lacy had been separated from her ex-husband for a little over three years; this would be her third year hosting Thanksgiving. Two group members, Linda and Carla, said they would be thrilled to join her. They were about the same age as Lacy and delighted in the idea that they would be spending time with her for their first Thanksgiving since divorcing. About a week after Thanksgiving, when group resumed, Linda and Carla excitingly insisted that Lacy tell the group members a story that she had shared with them during Thanksgiving dinner. Immediately, without hesitation, Lacy began to tell the story.

Lacy told us that during her first Thanksgiving after separating, she had three girlfriends over for dinner. When she took the turkey out of the oven, her friends were aghast. "My gosh, Lacy, what did you do to that turkey?" Lacy's response was, "Whatever do you mean? That turkey is cooked perfectly." They pointed to the rear portion of the turkey, where it looked like about three inches had been raggedly cut off and were missing. Lacy explained, "You have to cut about three inches off the back of a turkey before you cook it. My mother taught me to do that." Her guests could not let that go and insisted on a more thorough explanation.

Lacy offered to ask her mother, who lived in another state, and her three friends encouraged her to call right then. Lacy telephoned her mother, who said, "Lacy, that's just the way you do it. Ask your grandmother. She can explain it better than me." Again, her friends pressed for more of an explanation and insisted that she call her grandmother, who lived in an assisted living facility. Lacy called and her grandmother came to the phone. Lacy explained to her grandmother that her friends did not understand why she had to cut about three inches off the back of the turkey before cooking it, and that her mother could not explain it to their satisfaction. Lacy's grandmother laughed and laughed. Lacy pressed her, "Grandma, why?" Grandmother then responded in a sarcastic voice, "Lacy, you are so silly. The reason I cut a few inches off the back end of a turkey before cooking it was because I never had a pan big enough."

The "turkey story" promoted several enthusiastic group discussions. There were insights about our families of origin, and how we learn things that were once useful or even essential for survival in the past. I have come to understand that in every culture and in every family, over the generations, there are behaviors and beliefs that become outdated and unnecessary, borne out of a time when conformity was a function of necessity, security, and even survival. Yet those behaviors and beliefs often continue long after their purpose and usefulness have expired. Families are systems that teach us rules and roles; and outdated rules and roles can continue to be passed on for generations, impacting our behaviors, beliefs, and choices—as detailed in *Peoplemaking* (Satir 1972).

It also has become clear to me that clients have their own unique ways of communicating. I have come to recognize that every client "brings their family with them" to each session, and that understanding their family system is vital to good clinical work. A thorough client history, family history, and cultural assessment are critical to understanding a client's issues. Change processes that do not fit with the client's philosophy of how change occurs for them are not effective. Part of any assessment needs to include patterns and styles of communication, including non-verbal communication behaviors.

Lacy's high-context, metaphorical communication and some of her beliefs might seem unusual, such as divining with a stick for water on her property or being influenced by the spirits of deceased relatives; but they are accepted in her Appalachian culture. The therapist who originally referred her to my group had diagnosed Lacy with schizotypal personality disorder, which features odd beliefs and thinking, unusual perceptions and speech, and behavior that is odd, eccentric, or peculiar. In making the diagnosis, the clinician misunderstood Lacy's culture and its influence on her beliefs, thinking, and speech.

Cautions Around Assumptions, Constructs, and the Words We Use

Clients have taught me that—just as culture cannot be easily defined in terms of ethnicity, race, or country of origin— "family" is also not easily defined. Integral to many families, much more so than friends or neighbors, are "fictive kin." Discussed in detail in Chapter 6, these pseudo-family members can provide significance to the family structure and family functioning, impacting the family's ability to safely and sanely exist. Just as we cannot take anything for granted about the family's culture, we cannot take anything for granted about who the family members are and what constitutes the family hierarchy. Additionally, we cannot take for granted the family's values and beliefs. Family values vary broadly; although my clients who were parents almost universally expressed a desire that their children would have a better life with more opportunities, fulfillment, love, and amenities than they were able to achieve for themselves.

Choice of words is an important consideration for therapists. Neurolinguistic studies have made it clear that the words we use matter. I have learned not to ask "why," because it is often taken as judgmental or critical. When a family member shares a value, behavior, or belief that I need to understand at a deeper level, I find that asking a form of "How come?" is a more acceptable and less threatening approach than asking "Why?" I might ask, "How come you decided to do that?" or, "How did you come to decide that?" The language we use can help make or break our relationship with clients, so it is important that we choose words and sequences that are both respectful and empowering. Using the client's exact words will yield better results than using our clinical nomenclature, especially when defining the problem or setting goals.

Adult Children of Alcoholics and Inner Child Work

Several of the members in my groups for divorcing clients had been attending Al Anon self-help groups for many years. They were initially attracted to Al Anon because their spouse had a substance use disorder that had been affecting their marriage. Many of them had grown up in addictive family systems, with one or both parents addicted to alcohol or drugs. They found wisdom in the Al Anon language, stories, and information about addiction and codependency.

Among themselves, they shared their "recovering" experiences; and in group, they expressed insightful ideas as they attempted to better understand their feelings, tendencies, and choices.

The profound effect our families of origin can have on us is illustrated through the "adult children of alcoholics" (ACOA) literature on treatment ideas and concepts. In the 1980s and 1990s, there were books published and workshops designed to address the impact of "addictive family systems" or other dysfunctional family dynamics on children and "adult children." Group members were able to identify feelings and behaviors in common with those referenced in books as exhibited by ACOAs. It was enlightening and empowering for them to have a context in which to better understand themselves.

In Chapter 5, we briefly introduced the concept of the "inner child" as a strategy to connect with emotional pain that originated in childhood. ACOA clients had refined "inner child work" into a powerful, "hands-on" healing process to acknowledge the pain of your child within—literally the child you once were—and to comfort that child within who feels pain, fear, anger, or whatever unresolved feelings and issues might exist. Many clients symbolically postured as if holding a baby or small child, sometimes with rocking motions, and self-talked words of comfort. Some of the processes at times resembled the Gestalt therapy dynamics of using an empty chair to represent a person or issue. Most of those clients, in one way or another, expressed a belief that they could now self-protect and stated that they no longer felt vulnerable.

The physical act of self-comfort and caring by symbolically taking active control and nurturing oneself quickly fostered emotional and behavioral changes. Inner child work looked to be significantly more effective than other self-care methods commonly prescribed at the time, such as affirmations or self-talk. Clients practicing inner child self-nurturing believed that they had the ability to comfort and even heal themselves. It was clear to me that when the "problem was perceived as 'inside' of oneself," it was more difficult to resolve than when it could be put in front of the client and held, talked to, or managed—even if only symbolically. Meeting a client "where they are at" means that we need to acknowledge the issues they identify and what is working or not working for them.

Inner child work was not a process that I taught or was teaching my clients. It was a personal solution that several clients found workable and effective on their own. Clients discussed it and practiced it outside of my therapy groups, and then sometimes shared their self-nurturing experiences with the group. Exception questions such as, "When do you feel in control, resolved, soothed, freed from the trauma of the past, and more healed and empowered?" yielded descriptions of the inner child process. It was not a harmful practice and in fact helped facilitate desired outcomes. Clients who were recently separated or divorced and grieving were able to better connect with others and felt supported and understood. In solution work, we learn from clients what works for them and to assess progress or a lack thereof. There was no doubt that the self-nurturing processes were impacting more than a handful of clients in a positive, empowering way. And it was a practice that kept them in the present with their feelings and behaviors. Clients focused on themselves and believed that their parents had done the best they could.

Group Work is Not for All Clients or Therapists

Children who grow up with a parent who has a compulsion or addiction are often susceptible to the effects of trauma stemming from family of origin dynamics. We need to keep in mind that the compulsive catalyst does not have to be alcohol: it could be substance use, work, sexual addiction, compulsive spending, depression, and more. Children in addictive/compulsive family systems acquire roles to help rescue, cover up for, and preserve the family. We do not lose those childhood roles just because we grow into adulthood. Seeing our adult decisions and behaviors in the context of family dynamics can be a step toward self-understanding and even forgiveness for some. At the same time, we need to acknowledge that our childhood roles are not chains that prevent us from growth and healing. We acquire strengths beyond survival skills from our childhood experiences; and those strengths allow us to chart and live our chosen path if we work in that direction.

Clients in my practice who identified as ACOAs reinforced the idea that even though we do not have to know the reasons for a behavior in order to extinguish it, it can be reassuring to understand the role we played in our family of origin. Clients appreciated making sense of their vulnerabilities as adults to assume the posture, role, and behaviors from childhood at their workplace or in close relationships. There is something emotionally empowering about understanding family of origin dynamics—not to blame, but for clarity. Most of my clients let go of wondering why their parents "did what they did," and expressed a thirst for learning more about family dynamics and the roles they and their siblings played to preserve the family. Knowing that susceptibilities were tendencies, not chains, opened the door for them to exert free will and personal power.

One of the tragedies that can occur from misguided family of origin work is that clients can build anger and resentment over a lifetime. Wendy, a client who was referred from another therapist, was consumed by anger and even hate toward her mother. She ranted about how her mother had mistreated her and blamed her mother for adult problems from multiple marriages to a sleep disorder to interpersonal conflicts at work. I had learned through some uncomfortable experiences to require that all clients attend several individual therapy sessions with me before deciding whether to admit them into a group. Wendy attended three individual sessions in three weeks; and although we were able to process exception and coping questions, she returned to each of the next sessions with vitriol toward her mother and complaints about how miserable her life had become.

Clients in the grip of anger and resentment from their past can bring a counterproductive tone into group. Clearly, Wendy was not ready for group. And my concern was duly for the clients in group and their clinical work. Likely, Wendy would have used her time in group to vent about her mother without finding resolution. More than five previous years of therapy directed at how her mother was unfit and cruel led Wendy to conclude with conviction that her mother alone was responsible for all of her problems, failings, and emotional issues. She was consumed, almost in a cult-like state, about how her mother could have been so uncaring and brutal. Her pain was heart-wrenching. It was unnerving and emotionally painful for me whenever a client was overcome by trauma and a therapist had stoked that pain rather than working toward resolution for the client.

Solution work with Wendy, individually over time, could have opened the door to other possibilities; but her conviction was to continue individual sessions with her other therapist. I was sad for Wendy and the choice she made. I knew that I could have helped her to let go and move into a comforting set of solutions that she would eventually identify. But as a client-need-driven, solution therapist, I understood that I was not the expert on her domain, and her choice would serve her in a way that must have fit for her at that time. Her agenda was about expressing and feeling her anger, not working at healing her pain or letting go of her hurt and anger. I can only hope that when she was ready to heal her pain, Wendy would find a therapist who was helpful. She never returned to take that step with me.

There are many complications in facilitating therapy groups that can result in emotional harm. When I began group work with clients, I was not totally aware of the risks and complications. Over time, I began to recognize the need for boundaries among clients in group and ways to reduce some of the risks; but there are things we cannot control. Screening potential group members might help, but it will not eliminate many of those risks. For example, group members could become a social cluster and meet outside of group. Some group members will be vulnerable to romantic involvements. There are strong possibilities for alliances, triangulation, scapegoating, and breaches of confidentiality—especially when group members might have common acquaintances or friends outside of group. Resentments can fester. Jealousies might smolder. Anger could erupt.

Therapists need to recognize what they can do to make groups more functional, meaningful, secure, and safe for group members. We need to maintain control of the group process and set ground rules. It is essential to screen members for entry and retain the right to discharge group members. Some important provisions can be accomplished partially through informed consent; although it can be challenging, for example, to ban group members from relationships or social outings. Therapists also need to be cautious about seeing clients in individual or couples therapy while they are group members. Maintaining confidentiality in individual work is an important consideration; yet a therapist is put in a horrible predicament when a client says, "I don't want my group to know that I was forced to be an undercover informant for the police and my work resulted in Jack's brother getting busted."

In spite of the exercise of caution, I came to understand the reasons that spouses or members of a couple cannot receive group services from one therapist, even in separate groups. Jill had been attending one of my groups for several months when she introduced her fiancé, Chad, to me. Chad expressed an interest in attending group with her, identifying with issues that we were addressing such as recovery from divorce and loss, dysfunctional family of origin issues, and challenges with getting close to others. After several individual sessions with Chad, I told him that he was welcome to attend group, but not the same group as Jill. His response was, "I just want to talk about and resolve my stuff or I'll never get it right in a relationship. It's fine. Any group that will help me with Jill will be great."

Chad sounded like a good candidate, so I put him into the other group from Jill's. Then one day in group, I heard Jill say:

> I am just so lucky to be engaged to Chad. Every man I've ever been with has cheated on me. Chad has always been faithful. He's not the cheating kind. I know this relationship will work. I can trust him.

A couple of weeks later, I heard Chad say in his group:

> I've been told I have a problem with intimacy. I guess I do. I have to lie a lot to cover my tracks, if you know what I mean. I've always cheated in

> every relationship. I even cheated in this one, on Jill, the first week she
> moved in with me. I don't know why. I guess I'm just a prick.

I cringed. This was a disaster just waiting to happen. I could not legally
tell Jill; but keeping this secret was unethical and potentially harmful.
Fortunately for me, the group spent a lot of energy intervening with Chad
to "come clean" with Jill if he really wanted a lasting, authentic relationship. He talked to her about his history of infidelity and his one-time
affair while they were involved. She broke off the relationship and he
quit group.

More than ten years later, I was investigating a complaint for the
board of examiners for alcohol, drug, and gambling counselors.
Coincidentally, the therapist who was the subject of the complaint was
facilitating two groups in his practice, and had one member of a couple
in one group and the second member in the other group. The female
group member had told her group that fidelity was important to her,
and she was confident her partner was faithful. The male told his group
that he was a sex addict and liked to "play around." Understandably,
the therapist, hearing both disclosures, was disturbed—as I had been
years before under similar circumstances. One major difference for that
therapist was that the male client's group was not proactive, and the
majority of the group members did not encourage him to disclose his
infidelity to his partner.

The therapist who was the subject of the complaint was concurrently
providing individual therapy to the female client and decided to address
this issue with her in their next session. Trying to do what he perceived
to be the right thing, he asked if her boyfriend was faithful. When she
answered in the affirmative, he tried to "tease" some doubt out of her with
comments such as:

> How can you know? Are you certain? If it's important to you, you need
> to really take a hard look and verify that he is faithful. We both know
> a lot of women are naïve about men being unfaithful, so you need to
> be sure.

The therapist's intentions may have been good, but his strategy to correct
the problem was disastrous.

Naturally, the questioning made her suspicious; and although the therapist tried to pass off his comments and questions as protective and routine,
she knew something was up. Confronting her boyfriend and continuing to
check on him, she deduced that her suspicions were probably warranted.
Ultimately, he admitted that he had not been faithful, and they broke
up. Each filed a complaint against the therapist with the licensing board,

and the male filed an additional complaint alleging that the therapist had violated his right to confidentiality. Reading the complaints made it crystal clear that I had truly "dodged a bullet" years before.

Earlier in this chapter, I stated that therapists need to be cautious about seeing clients in individual or couples therapy while they are group members. My takeaway from this investigation was that it is not prudent for a therapist to concurrently have clients who are a couple in individual or group therapy, even if they are in separate groups. In Chapter 12, I detail that in couples and marriage therapy, the relationship is the client, and discuss some of the "beartraps" when we attempt to work with those clients outside of a couples session.

Childhood Roles Can Spill Over into Adulthood

Publications such as *Adult Children of Alcoholics* provided explanations for the feelings and behaviors experienced by children, teens, and adults who grew up with a parent who had an addiction or compulsion (Woititz 1983). The literature hypothesizes that ACOAs, and adult children of compulsive parents, more so than most, have tendencies to become isolated; fear authority figures; seek approval; be frightened by angry people; be terrified of personal criticism; become alcoholics/compulsives themselves, marry them, or both; view life as victims; and act overly responsible or punish themselves for not being responsible enough. They can also be more concerned with others than themselves; have difficulty completing projects; exhibit "black and white" thinking; find it difficult to have fun; and judge themselves harshly.

Accordingly, many clinicians recognize that the roles we play as children in our family can also have strong—sometimes beneficial—influences on our adult lives and careers. Although there may be some minor differences in the literature, most authors express similar ideas about the effects on those who grow up in homes with an addictive parent. "Heroes" can be super responsible and dependable—qualities that help them to succeed as leaders and managers; but they can also be rigid, controlling, and judgmental. "Scapegoats" are often generous, sensitive, and compassionate, supporting the "underdog" and rescuing the disadvantaged; however, they can tend to put others first, make poor choices for themselves, and violate rules in order to rescue or protect other people. "Mascots" commonly have qualities that enable them to be entertainers, perhaps as actors or comedians; and they find it easy to give love to others, but are challenged to feel worthy and receive love. "Lost children" often seek quiet jobs that will keep them in the background, such as in accounting, and are prone to be exacting and careful; but, at the same time they are shy, withdrawn, and socially isolated.

Self-help books such as *A Guide for Adult Children of Alcoholics* are often rich in concepts that promote self-understanding and ideas for acceptance, forgiveness, and healing (Gravitz and Bowden 1983); but there are significant cautions that must be considered before we attempt to apply these concepts to others and ourselves. We are unique and experience a variety of "outlier" circumstances throughout our lives. We are much more than our experiences and circumstances, so it is important that we do not stereotype or predict a client's future. There are variabilities in genetics, life experiences, connections, and system dynamics. Deaths, births, stepparents, extended families, individual personalities, personal influences, distractions, and interventions—including contacts with teachers, school counselors, therapists, peer groups, coaches, and dance teachers—all make a difference in our childhood development. Generational, cultural, and socioeconomic factors contribute to the development of our belief systems, personality development, and choices. Abuse, neglect, abandonment, and victimization can set us back, cause lasting emotional harm; or can plant the seeds of resilience. There are no crystal balls in therapy.

References

Gravitz, H. L., and Bowden, J. D. (1983). *A Guide for Adult Children of Alcoholics.* New York: Simon & Schuster, Inc.

Satir, V. (1972). *Peoplemaking.* Palo Alto, CA: Science and Behavior Books, Inc.

Woititz, J. G. (1983). *Adult Children of Alcoholics.* Deerfield Beach, FL: Health Communications Inc.

10 A Family from the Philippines

Every Family Has Its Own Unique Culture

Decades of facilitating interactive workshops on culture and diversity have led me to conclude that many clinicians misunderstand both the concepts of and the interplay between "culture" and "diversity." I teach that the best working definition of "culture" is: "Culture is much more than race, ethnicity, and country of origin. There is diversity in every culture and every family has its own unique culture." It is concerning when well-meaning clinicians unwittingly stereotype client families, improperly apply assessment and diagnostic criteria, or interpret results from evaluation and testing without taking into account cultural differences in family structure, communication, codes of conduct, beliefs, and dynamics. Human beings tend to be ethnocentric, at least to some extent, believing their own "culture" to be superior. There are many societies where a plurality would believe it beneficial for everyone to conform to their culture, or at least aspects of their culture. Boris Bizumic (2018) takes an interesting look at ethnocentrism as a social, psychological, and attitudinal construct.

Culturally competent interventions would include the completion of a thorough history and cultural assessment early in treatment. Culture impacts many things, including rules, roles, norms, beliefs, communication, and philosophy of change. Best practice clinical work requires an understanding of a client's history, culture, strengths, life experiences, definition of the problem, and goals as a prerequisite to formulating a treatment plan. In order to engage a client effectively in the therapeutic process, we must first learn about the client's "philosophy of change"; recognize the strengths of the client and the client's family; accept the client's style of communication; prioritize the client's agenda; respect the client as an expert; and employ a methodology that is compatible with the family structure and hierarchy.

DOI: 10.4324/9781003397380-10

Values and Codes of Conduct

Geographical, religious, and social factors can affect and even alter family culture. When assessing a family's culture, in addition to the family dynamics, rules, hierarchy, and behaviors, we need to consider geographical, religious, and social factors adopted by the family. Assessment also necessitates an understanding of a family's values and codes of conduct. "Values" are strongly held beliefs influenced by historical experiences, and are often similar across cultures—for example, life is valued, and homicide is considered a crime in most cultures. "Codes of conduct" encourage behaviors that are consistent with accepted values. Values are hierarchical and sometimes compete. Over generations, circumstances can alter the position of competing values in the hierarchy.

Looking back, I can reflect on parts of my own culture and how my personal cultural experience tarnished my objectivity early in my counseling career. My grandparents—socioeconomically poor immigrants who lived in Brooklyn tenements and suffered discrimination—built their hope for the future on their children and grandchildren completing advanced education and attaining a profession where they would be independent and not have to rely on others for employment. Education was a dominant value and believed to be the solution for improving the future for children. Without recognizing the connection, when I began working at the Welfare Division with a population of "Children in Need of Supervision" status children and families (see Chapter 4), I erred by encouraging the parents to go back to school and complete their education, sometimes offering it as a treatment plan goal. These were my values; but they were not necessarily the values and priorities of my clients, who were facing serious life issues at the time.

In addition to the next generations of children in my family completing their education and attaining a profession, other dominant values in my family were built on the belief that extended family was important and that we all needed to live close to one another. I can recall as a child that we had dozens of relatives living in tenements within four blocks of each other. We needed help and support from one another. Our wellbeing—even our survival—depended on it. Ironically, children becoming educated and attaining professional licensure meant that there were important job opportunities with higher standards of living some distance from the tenements where other family members lived. Survival was no longer dependent on family members living physically close to each other. One by one, younger adult relatives moved away to enjoy a higher standard of living. The transition was not easy and there were hurt feelings—primarily among the grandparents, aunts, and uncles who had made educational opportunities possible for their children and grandchildren.

Family members maintained close ties, but now from a distance. Family was a central value and still important; but for this next generation, the nuclear family, education, attaining a profession, and succeeding were higher in the values hierarchy compared with living physically close to extended family. In my work with families, I have seen similar dynamics where competing values would lead to crises that had multi-generational implications. I have learned from client-families to be sensitive to their cultures and their hierarchy of needs. Additionally, their disclosures have helped me to gain insight into my own family dynamics.

Intervention With a First-Generation Family from the Philippines

This story of an intervention with a first-generation family from the Philippines vividly illustrates the need to understand and work congruently among the interplay between family structure and hierarchy; family dynamics; culture, cultural divides, and cultural transitions; competing values and codes of conduct; client agendas and agency agendas; and family history. Hearing a family's journey and understanding their struggles require a clinician to be deeply empathic and accepting.

At the time of referral, the family consisted of the father; the mother; three daughters aged 17, 15 and 13; and a six-year-old son. The children appeared well adjusted, were good students with close friendships, and were observed to be respectful and compliant with their parents' requests. The mother and father had left the Philippines for the United States 17 years earlier, just before the birth of their first child. Their maternal and paternal extended family remained in the Philippines and had severed all contact with them.

The 17-year-old girl was a high-school senior, and the alleged child abuse had occurred when the girl had attempted to leave the house one evening around 10:00 p.m. to see friends, against her father's wishes. Her father physically restrained her at the door and during the struggle she bruised her face when he held her against the wall. A school counselor reported the bruise to Child Protective Services (CPS). CPS assessed this as high risk because during their investigation, the mother and girls would not answer questions without first looking to the father for his consent; and often he gave the answers instead of waiting for them to speak. The conclusion from the CPS assessment team and collateral agencies was that the father must be very controlling, the mother and children must be afraid of him, and there was a strong potential for more serious violence. The father was arrested and forced to leave the house; the law enforcement report and the district attorney described him as a violent man who likely abused his wife and children. The agencies involved proposed that he be required to complete a full program for domestic violence offenders.

The CPS worker had asked for a psychosocial family assessment and psychological evaluations to explore family issues, patterns of domestic violence, and emotional trauma of family members living in the household. Her stated goal was to determine what services might reduce the risk and help the mother and children stay safe. During the initial assessment by CPS, it was concluded that the father was only marginally cooperative, although he professed strong love and dedication to his family while denying that he was violent. Family members were somewhat reluctant to fully participate in interviews without the father present. They denied that there had been any prior "abuse," although each (including the father) readily admitted to all the details of the recent incident. The father and the other family members insisted—even begged—that the father be allowed to move back home.

The psychological assessment found the father cooperative but not willing to take responsibility for wrongdoing or engage in "significant conversation about other family members" without his family present. The report documented from several sources the "profile of a domestic violence family," and stated that this family was consistent with that profile. The mother and children did not see anything wrong with the father's physical restraint of the girl; and the "abused" daughter called it "my father's responsibility" because, she explained, "I was willfully disobedient." When asked, "What is important to you and what would you like to have happen?" the father responded: "For all of us to be together and for my wife and me to talk better."

The report concluded that all the family members expressed that they felt safe around dad, and continued:

> although there are not allegations of abuse against the other children or spouse, this must be considered high risk. There must be fear and apprehension that the children are not admitting. We do not recommend that (the father) return home without a safety plan, in-home services, and consistent monitoring, if at all.

Based partially on this psychological report, the CPS worker referred the family to an in-home family therapist provided through a community resource center. The plan was for the father to attend in-home family sessions and only be allowed to move back home after the in-home therapist and CPS had developed a safety plan, and Child Welfare had agreed that it would be safe.

A couple of weeks later, during a case staffing meeting, the in-home therapist asked for help because she was unsure of the effectiveness of her intervention. The community resource center asked me to meet with the family to help provide whatever was needed. I agreed to team with the in-home therapist and the CPS worker to provide family therapy in order to reduce risk and strengthen family functioning. The CPS worker, assessment coordinator, psychologist, and in-home therapist were all female. I was the first male in the "system," other than the arresting police officer, to address the father in his home.

There are two important points that must be made here. First, we need to accept that these were good people trying to protect children and bring the appropriate services to the family. Whether or not they were culturally competent or made sound judgments should not cancel their good intentions and mission-driven protection of children. The second thing is to acknowledge that the family's culture is their own, and to be cautious not to stereotype Filipinos or any other group. Acknowledging that diversity exists within every culture, and that each family has its own unique culture, literally means that we must begin from scratch and assess every family as a unique, standalone culture.

I began my intervention by first meeting with the CPS worker and in-home therapist, getting a thorough "play-by-play" from the start of their involvement. We worked out ground rules that would enable me to be the primary therapist and remain independent as the family's therapist, while also allowing them to continue their supportive, assessment, advocacy, and protective roles. As part of my assessment to better understand the situation prior to meeting the family, I asked each agency participant: "What was good about the intervention? What concerns do you have about it?"

Just prior to my first session with the family, I asked the in-home therapist: "What are the strengths of each of the family members? What compliments might you offer them?" I also asked her to share those strengths and compliments with the family as part of her introduction of me at the initial session. I made it clear that I would only accept the referral if the family was in charge of accepting or rejecting my help, without consequences; and I would ask them to allow me three meetings in their home before making that decision.

My strategy was to engage and join with the family during the first session or two—employing standard Rogerian ideas around listening and respecting the family's point of view—and to empathetically review with them what I had been told. I was particularly interested in hearing their responses to my summary of what I had been told, especially after all the difficulties they had been through. Validating their point of view would be important if we were going to begin in a positive place. I also made it clear that they were the experts on their own family, and I needed to learn from them what they wanted to accomplish while working with me.

I knew that it would be critical in the first session to learn of the family's primary "agenda" and the father's primary "agenda," and to clearly indicate that I respected their ideas. From the history I had been provided, it became clear that the father was the family patriarch, and my hypothesis was that most likely change would come through him first. I would test that theory in the first session and confirm that it was true. It became clear almost immediately that assigning a male therapist who was a husband and father would open doors to disclosure and trust that had not been available previously.

The father asked me several questions about myself and seemed interested in my marital status and family. He then began to inquire if I knew about communication between husbands and wives. (It is probable that he was checking to see if I was qualified to address his issues.) This discussion (which revealed his agenda) led to a revelation that he and his wife had had "communication" difficulties for several years, and fortunately I was able to normalize and validate some of their issues. Most impactful was the revelation that he and his wife were from different tribes in the Philippines; that their families of origin actually spoke different dialects (in addition to Tagalog, which they spoke in common); that they had married against their respective parents' wishes, which is why they had left the Philippines; that their families of origin had presented cultural conflicts that they had never fully reconciled; and that they did not understand many aspects of what they called "American culture."

It was significant to learn that their tribal families in the Philippines could never have forgiven them for marrying outside of their tribes, so they were ostracized. Both mother and father described being ostracized by their parents and siblings as the most hurtful thing that they had ever experienced. One of the things that their parents' culture had in common was that families were patriarchal in nature, with the father having almost absolute authority over the children, including the use of physical control. Mother was very supportive of father's authority and actions. But there were also significant tribal differences that had manifested under the surface and caused previously unspoken tensions between them.

It was clear that the family and father's agenda was for the father to return home and for Child Welfare to close the case. But notably, the father also had another agenda, which had been his primary agenda for many years—even before the involvement of Child Welfare. He wanted communication with his wife about family issues, rules, and problems to be open, and for her to let him know what she would like to have happen when issues between them about the children arose. His tribal culture gave shared authority to the mother when it came to issues regarding the children. The rules and roles of her culture demanded that a wife defer to her husband any discussion or decision-making regarding family matters. Candid, open discussions about family matters in front of the children or about the children inside the family home would not be acceptable in her family of origin. Her upbringing had been strong and stern about a wife's role, and what was permissible for a wife to do or say in the family home.

Understanding the rules and dynamics, I began asking about exceptions to the communication difficulties with his wife. ("When is it you and your wife have been able to talk about issues, maybe a little bit—sharing ideas and concerns together?") It was clear from their answers that nowhere in the house or in the children's presence were they able to communicate "as parenting equals." I insisted that there must have been a time and place where it had happened, even once, just a little bit—a time when they had been able to speak interactively and openly about family matters, including the children. What we found out was remarkable. They only had one car, and the wife drove her husband to and from work every day. Inside the car, while she was driving, they were sometimes able to speak "as equals" about family matters. Without realizing it, they already had their solution—they just did not have the awareness of how to put it into use more constructively.

Now I knew that there was the potential for parental discussions and solution building within the confines of the car if the wife was driving. From their disclosure, it was obvious that in the past, those discussions had occurred only sporadically and spontaneously during tense times, and thus were often less than productive. I surmised that unless they could have discussions whenever needed, issues would probably not be addressed in a timely and constructive manner. So, their "homework" was to go for a drive anytime one or both needed to talk. We agreed on some ground rules. "Anytime" meant literally anytime. Either could request a drive together and it had to be honored. "Mother keeps the keys and drives." It worked!

Communication difficulties with his wife and concerns about the children were two of several issues that the father could not have discussed with a female worker alone. I continued to team with both the in-home therapist and the CPS worker during home visits, so that a male was included in all discussions from that point on. We were able to communicate American "taboos," such as physical abuse of children and the legal definition of "physical abuse," which made the reason behind the intervention by CPS a little more understandable for the family. But even so, the vulnerable issue for this family was the clash between the father's duty to discipline children for what outsiders might consider to be typical teenage behavior, and the laws limiting the extent of physical discipline. In other words, the clash between the father's culture and child-rearing practices in the United States still caused him strife and significant concern. It seemed to him that he was not able to do the right thing for his children.

It was incumbent on us—professionals and family members alike—to find a way to respect the parents' customs and authority, while supporting safe solutions to allow the children enough space to fit in with their peers in America. We had already seen what could happen when the parents' pressure to maintain cultural parenting traditions clashed with a child's need to be a teenager and meet with friends. And, perhaps ironically, it was clear that the children expected—even insisted—that the parents remain true to what a parent in authority who loved their children must do. Each of the children supported their parents' right to use any means to physically restrain a "willfully disobedient" child. On the other hand, peer relationships are also important to children, especially teenagers. We needed a breakthrough moment in therapy, and it happened after a couple more sessions.

Some of our discussions after the third therapy session involved the parenting of the children; dreams and hopes for the children; and some of the differences that mom and dad had experienced in their families of origin at different stages of their own childhood. We were able to transition so that we could concurrently address some of the parents' struggles with issues that originated with their own families of origin, while helping them to construct solutions to address or even resolve the spillovers that had been negatively impacting their marital relationship. The father became emotional during a discussion of how their families of origin had been intolerant of their marital engagement and choices. Their families of origin had made it impossible for them to be married and remain in the Philippines. Each parent professed strong love for the other and reaffirmed their absolute need to leave the Philippines in order to live their own lives. Remaining in the Philippines would have made it impossible for them to enjoy life as a couple and as parents. Although they still carried a great deal of sadness over losing their families, neither had any regrets about their decisions.

I was processing a series of questions with the parents about their love for their children. They brought up their duty to protect the children, so I asked, "What will you be doing to protect your children from the kind of trauma and hurt that you experienced?" Apparently, the parents did not fully understand the intent of my question and strayed from the content, talking about their role as protectors and that the children had to follow their rules. I acknowledged that their standard was for the children to abide by their wishes, in all cases. The father said that this was essential, for their own sake, if they were to live in his house or even be a part of his family.

Noting the father's reaction, I saw the opportunity to ask him an empathy question that happened to open the door for a significant breakthrough: "I guess that I'm wondering if you are saying that this is the way it is in your family; that in each generation, children will have to move far away from their parents to live their own lives?" After a very brief silence, the father began to sob, realizing that he was doing something similar to his children to what his parents and in-laws had done to him and his wife. He continued to sob and his wife began to cry also, overwhelmed by grief and empathy for their children. I was overcome by their reaction, as was the in-home therapist; and we teared up in sympathy with them.

The parents thereafter took a different direction in therapy. They asked about American children, their friendships, what they want, and what they need to be happy. They wanted to know how to be proper parents for their children to be successful, happy, and respectful at the same time. My response was that I was not the best expert on American children and teens, but that they had four experts in the house. We included the children in the remaining sessions, and it was evident that the structure of this family was reshaped to accommodate the needs and ideas of the children. We addressed the children's need to be respectful of their father, while still functioning as American children or teens. We supported the parents in retaining their authority as parents and complimented their willingness to hear and consider the reasonable needs of their children. And of course, we continued to help the couple resolve longstanding differences that originated from their tribes.

One question I have been asked about the decision to include the children: "Were you comfortable involving the six-year-old in the sessions?" The answer is that the six-year-old (he turned seven during the intervention), as a male, had a higher "status" in the family than the girls and was an integral part of the change that was evolving. He was intelligent and mature beyond his years. There was never anything discussed that concerned me about his presence.

As it turned out, this father was gentle, honest, and sincere. And all members were closely bonded. It would have been "disgraceful" for the father not to use physical means to control his children if they were "willfully disobedient" according to the parent's culture and family rules; and the children would have lost respect for him if he had not showed proper authority based on the values with which they had been raised. But now there was room for this family to thrive within two cultures.

A big part of our intervention was to advocate for the family in the larger system and convince the courts to not pursue the original punitive course of action. We addressed with CPS the fact that the father was very caring and wanted to protect and nurture his children. The children could not be any safer. All the children had attractive personalities and were high achievers in school, with glowing self-respect and confidence. There was no significant risk of abuse. The original incident was a result of the father blocking his daughter from leaving the house against his wishes—there was no malice, temper, or hitting—and the circumstances around the incident had been resolved. This was a fully cooperating, functional family!

The parents had us schedule afternoon sessions so that they would end around 5:00 p.m. in order to accommodate their dinner customs when guests were in their home. We "had to attend" several family dinners as part of their way of connecting with and embracing us. Watching this family at dinner and after dinner was enjoyable. They were loving, inter-active, and close. In appreciation, we were invited to a wonderful dinner party at case closure, where they talked about and celebrated their family blessings.

CPS, while attempting to protect these children, misunderstood the issues and made errors because an accurate cultural and family assessment was not completed as a part of the initial contacts with this family. The psychologist erred by failing to consider culture and language when interpreting the results of a standardized assessment and clinical inter-view. Additionally, the courts did not adequately question the submissions of the agencies and professionals involved with the investigation and assessment. The family ultimately responded to the intervention because they were respected; their "agenda" was acknowledged and met; their cul-ture was understood and accepted; and they were consulted through a non-blaming, collaborative, strength-based approach.

There is much that we learned from this family beyond what we knew about the fundamentals of culture and family structure. This experi-ence taught us that understanding the history of a family's culture, over generations, might provide ideas for a richer intervention and solutions. We also came to better understand how clients can become disenfranchised and victimized when public agencies and the courts pigeonhole or stereotype behavior; and that assessment and testing without a proper understanding of cultural factors and family structure can be inept and destructive.

While we engaged and counseled the family from the Philippines, our office had been participating in an "in-house" research project. Sometimes, as a teaching tool, a "clinical autopsy" is performed when interventions are not successful. However, this was a successful intervention—so much so that we conducted a study of "what worked" for future reference and teaching. Here's what we identified:

- The family was approached at a time of crisis and was receptive to change after it was demonstrated that the intervention could be worthwhile.
- Engagement and joining resulted in an alliance with the family.
- The family's history and culture were assessed, understood, and respected, so that they felt respect and acceptance.
- The father was not the problem; the problem was the family's difficulty in resolving the dilemma of clashing cultures, and the legal system's failure to understand the family's culture.

- A male therapist was made available at a time when the family needed a male to help the father address certain issues.
- The family system was entered through the patriarch, respecting the family structure, roles, and rules.
- The father's "agenda" was understood and an exception to the parental communication problem was identified.
- The family's agenda was identified, and the clinician valued and communicated that they were on the same page.
- The family were complimented on their strengths and efforts.
- The family were respected as experts.
- Solutions were elicited—the family were not told or pressured to make changes.
- The clinicians empathized and sympathized with the family's dilemma and struggles.
- The family prioritized and identified the solutions.
- The clinicians respected the family's processes, priorities, and goals throughout the intervention.

A working clinical understanding of the family system would say that it primarily supports traditional values and behaviors, but can be repositioned to support change as well. The architects of systemic, structural, and strategic thinking in family therapy have contributed to our understanding of how values, rules, roles, relationships, and behaviors interplay. This family from the Philippines affirmed that in order to preserve their family system and relationships, and resolve "clashing cultures and subcultures," our intervention needed to proceed from the parental hierarchy down. My experience with this family, most importantly, demonstrated that when parents' love and empathy for their children can be enlisted, even seemingly rigid systems can bend.

Reference

Bizumic, B. (2018). *Ethnocentrism: Integrated Principles*. London: Routledge.

11 Intensive Family Services

Families with Challenges and Few Resources

As was discussed in Chapter 1, during the 1990s several highly skilled clinicians—including Insoo Kim Berg—became interested in working with families within the child welfare system. The foster care system was overwhelmed, and in 1993 Congress passed the Family Preservation and Support Act (PL103-66) to fund family support and in-home services for at-risk children and their families (Berg and Kelly 2000, p. 27). Historically, clinical work with Child Welfare clients had not produced desired outcomes, and many protective services' programs had been diverting funds for family mental health services into other programs. Insoo teamed with child welfare programs and their work showed promising results using SFBT supplemented with strategies to fit with child welfare protocols and families in the child welfare system. Berg and Kelly 2000). Federal grant monies were available for demonstration projects/research on SFBT with families at imminent risk of having their children placed into foster care. Clientele in the study featured families coerced into therapy who were not invested in treatment and did not trust the "system," but who would otherwise have had their children removed and placed into foster care.

As an early disciple of SFBT, I was hired as the clinical manager and regional research supervisor for this groundbreaking demonstration project to preserve and strengthen families in the child welfare system. Intensive Family Services (IFS) was a "clinical family support program" that provided intensive, in-home clinical and supportive services to families with a complexity of issues, and at imminent risk of having their children placed into therapeutic foster care. Research focused on family functioning and preservation, risk and safety, and behavioral health and addiction treatment, with service follow-up at three months, six months, and one year after case closure. Outcomes were highly successful and so a longitudinal study for up to ten years was added.

Clearly, the best outcome for a child is to see their family make positive changes to create a safe and nurturing experience for that child. The

DOI: 10.4324/9781003397380-11

state or county is not a good parent, regardless of whatever monies and resources are budgeted. Children need permanency; but during my tenure at IFS, it was not unusual for a foster child to experience three, five, even eight or more different foster homes despite agency efforts at permanency. Even under the best circumstances, outcomes for foster children are dicey. The jails, prisons, mental hospitals, and homeless are populated with children who were once in foster care. Crimes of trafficking, prostitution, and other forms of victimization are disproportionate among foster children (Hannan et al. 2017). Children separated from parents experience lifelong emotional trauma that manifests as attachment disorders, emotional disorders, and behavioral disorders. A recent quantitative review looking at 32 studies using the Preferred Reporting Items for Systematic Reviews and Meta-Analyses method showed clear but troubling results. Children who age out of the child welfare system "continue to struggle in all areas (education, employment, income, housing, health, substance abuse, and criminal involvement) compared to their peers in the general population" (Gypen et al. 2017, Abstract).

IFS's Interventions Had to Address a Plethora of Challenges

Studies and books about the plight of children after they leave foster care do not sufficiently paint the picture. The children's stories are real. The children are not words or numbers. They are victims of lifelong trauma and loss (Shirk, M. & Stangler, G. 2004). When I worked at Child Welfare, I saw those children and families. When I worked at Juvenile Justice, I saw those children and families. When I worked with children from charities or shelters, I saw those children. When I worked for the Department of Prisons, I saw those adult-children. When I worked at community treatment centers, I saw those adult-children who had come from the streets, or shelters, or correctional facilities. When I received funds from victims of crime programs to pay for therapy, I saw those adult-children who had run away or been taken and trafficked at a young age. At IFS, we intervened with children and families to reduce risk and improve family functioning so that those children would never have to go through the foster care system.

IFS staff keenly understood the consequences for children if intervention was not successful. In addition to allegations of child abuse or neglect, families receiving IFS services typically had multiple challenges to address, such as addiction, mental health, developmental disabilities, poverty, parenting deficits, child behavioral problems, and legal obligations. IFS had no authority to determine placement or remove children. Child Welfare staff maintained the responsibility for risk and safety determinations while the family received IFS in-home therapy.

It can be challenging to achieve a collaborative engagement with families in the child welfare system. Parents' initial reluctance to be vulnerable and completely honest was about protecting their family. As would be expected, their initial impression was that we were just another government program. By the time IFS received a referral, families were overwhelmed; had been threatened with or were experiencing significant legal consequences; lacked resources; had lost hope; were disempowered; and felt targeted and disrespected. The future both for the parents and for the children relied heavily on our ability to work effectively with the family. Family therapy was provided at least two days with four clinical hours per week in the family's home. IFS intervention was the last chance for the family to retain or regain physical and legal custody of their children.

The overall mission of IFS was to ensure safety first and, whenever possible, to facilitate a therapeutic intervention that would increase family functioning, cohesiveness, and capacity in order to preserve the family; build a safety net for parents and children; build on and improve parenting skills; mitigate issues of mental illness and addiction that negatively impacted risk or safety and parenting; bring resources and supports to the family that would help ensure continued progress beyond the term of IFS services; provide whatever assistance the children needed to be successful and emotionally healthy; help the family to make their home safe, nurturing, and loving; and team with the researchers in order to acquire or increase therapeutic skills and knowledge that could be applied to all Child Welfare family clientele.

The ideal outcome was to correct and strengthen the family for the child's sake—in other words, removing the risk from the family instead of removing the child. Solution-focused brief therapy (SFBT) began as the core approach; but as our research revealed new ideas and strategies, the model was supplemented with groundbreaking technologies in family assessment; goal setting; scaling; fast-forward, coping, and miracle question sequences; tasking; and metaphorical storytelling for psychoeducation that included parenting ideas and strategies. I was responsible for training staff, and developed a workshop based on our IFS clinical work with reluctant clients. The workshop was named "Brief Solution Oriented Family Therapy."

In all cases—regardless of culture, history, or presenting issues—research guidelines and best practice required us to respect the family as experts in their domain; elicit solutions from the family rather than telling the family what to do; engage the family around their solutions and assist them with tasks or resources to accomplish their goals connected to preserving their family; involve the whole family in the therapeutic process whenever possible; work toward helping the family to verbalize and visualize what might be possible; empower the family to protect their members and develop a safety plan; establish and build on what the family were customers over; respect and use the family's language; identify and employ the family's philosophy of change; and monitor and document the family's efforts and progress or challenges. We were tasked with maintaining allegiance to the SFBT approach, using recognized neurolinguistic language, question sequences, methods, and process work, plus compatible addendums that were shown to foster the collaborative alliance and enhance outcomes.

In-Home Family Therapy

We learned a great deal from our families, and the experiences we had with them taught us to be better in-home family therapists. Respecting the sanctity of a family's home was an important consideration. We asked permission to enter and then asked where the family would like us to sit. Inside their homes, we learned how they lived, what they treasured, how they coped, and what they wanted; and, perhaps most importantly, about their love for their children. As a group, the number one priority of the parents we encountered was for their children to have a better life than they did. Child Welfare staff may not have known that. Law enforcement may not have known that. Judges may not have known that. Coming from a place of respect and offering help without judgment opened the door for families to talk to us about what was important and meaningful for them.

IFS therapists practiced strict tenets of established family therapy that included seeing the whole family together in the home, sometimes including extended family. There were countless advantages to seeing a family in their natural environment. We were able to complete more accurate assessments; engage family members—even young children—in meaningful ways; reference family pictures or keepsakes during an intervention; more readily identify "hard service" needs and challenges; and note strengths and coping abilities. The family hierarchy was also more transparent within the family home versus a therapist's office.

Adolescent "Visitors" Such as Anna Became "Customers" of Family Therapy

Several therapists encountered situations where adolescent children would refuse to participate in family therapy. During one of my encounters as a co-therapist, I noticed that although the family's 15-year-old daughter, Anna, declined to sit in the living room and participate in family therapy, she left her bedroom door open and could hear everything. During each session, Anna would walk out of her room a couple of times past us to the kitchen, to get a beverage or just look in the refrigerator, and then return to her room.

I kept a file folder on my lap and recorded notes during each session; and as she slowly walked by from the kitchen to her bedroom, I noticed that Anna would stare at the notes on my lap, trying to read them. After a few sessions, I theorized that Anna was communicating to me that she was more than merely an eavesdropper, and might be receptive to joining in the therapeutic process with her family. What she needed from me was an opening to join with us on her terms to "save face."

I came up with an idea to engage her in a way that would not threaten her need to appear in control and independent. The next time Anna slowly walked by and tried to read the notes on my lap, I looked her in the eye, making it obvious that I had noticed. My hope was that she would say something to me. At first, she hesitated for a moment, quickly looking away, and then turned to walk to her room. About a minute, she came back and stood next to me. I continued to process a question with the family, writing a note during the exchange, and then looked up at her. After an awkward moment, Anna asked, "What are you writing?" I said:

Oh, I just keep track of what everyone says so that I can remember. I do it to try to be more helpful with your family. It's too difficult for me to try to remember everything without making notes. Here, you can see what I've written.

"I can?" she asked as I handed her the notes.

As she was looking over the notes, I said:

Anna, you know, you've given me a great idea. It's hard for me to write and talk at the same time. Could you do us a favor and help? Could you sit here and just write down for me what you hear that's important so that I can do better with the conversation?

Anna asked, "If you think I could do that, I guess. What do I write?" I said, "Whatever you hear that you think I need to remember." She agreed and took the pencil and papers as she pulled up a chair and sat down next to me.

Anna became more than a note taker, actively participating in the interaction for the remainder of the sessions. It turned out that she was the primary initiator of change in her family, and took an active role in proposing solutions and offering to complete tasks. Her family made significant strides in a relatively short time. Anna also did a great job taking notes and her handwriting was superb!

Assessment/Genograms

Our first 30 days of in-home clinical work with IFS families was considered the assessment period. We did both assessment and family therapy during that time, attempting to successfully join with and engage the family. On the 30th day, the family had to commit to continue services with us or find and secure services elsewhere to comply with their case plan. More than 90% of referred families accepted and completed the full term of IFS services. Our client-centered and family-centered practice philosophies were likely part of the reason for the high rate of acceptance; and the use of engaging assessment tools such as the genogram helped us to quickly collaborate and join with families.

A genogram is a diagram that illustrates several generations of family members, how they are related, and significant historical features or behaviors. Generations appear horizontally, one on top of the next, with relatives' names in circles connected by lines to indicate parents/ marriages/divorces across each generation. Children's names in circles appear below, connected by lines to the parents above and below to their children in the next generation, until several generations are illustrated. Then characteristics and issues are written next to each name—for example: "Uncle Bob; behavioral problems as child; dropped out of school 11th grade; alcoholic; seizure disorder; veteran Vietnam war; owned plumbing business; at age 45 stopped drinking and became dedicated AA member, well respected in his community." Families benefit from a visual history of multigenerational issues as well as family strengths and challenges, which can be helpful for building hope, self-understanding, and decisions for change.

When creating a genogram with families, we found it helpful to use a very large sheet of paper that covered their kitchen table. We included all family members as participants in creating the diagram. Young children were given crayons and allowed to draw in the margins of the document. Parents and older children were tasked with recording information using pencils (erasers were sometimes necessary) on the document as it was being developed through questions and discussions. When appropriate, parents were tasked with contacting a relative to clarify information, which often led to opportunities for extended family connections and even emotional or material support. The family was always provided with a copy of their genogram.

Families Challenged by Poverty and a Lack of Resources

My best guess is that 15% of our families would have been designated as living in multigenerational poverty. Another 10% to 20% may or may not have officially fallen below the designated poverty line, but their income was woefully inadequate. Parents of those low-income client families barely earned enough to provide even a basic standard of living despite working hard in full-time jobs and striving to make a better future for their children. Many had no other option but to rent homes or apartments in disrepair with tattered carpeting, cracked walls, and peeling paint. A number of families lived inside old school buses, fifth wheels, or trailers without electricity or running water. They might go to the "Y" to shower, use laundromats to clean their clothes, and dump trash in receptacles around the city.

We sat in their homes, on old, worn second or third-hand chairs and couches that had accumulated stains and dust over many decades; with flooring so tarnished that even a professional scrubbing would not have helped much. Vacuum cleaners and adequate cleaning supplies were considered luxuries, attainable only if sacrifices were made to their already scarce food and clothing budgets. Without cars or perhaps one "junky" car, some families had to live in neighborhoods that were within walking distance to work, markets, or schools. Somehow, they prepared adequate meals in dated kitchens with sinks, counters, and stoves too old for simple restoration. Yet there were family pictures on the wall; a table or area with the children's trophies and awards; and a corner set up for school study and homework.

Poverty demands thinking in the present as a means for survival and connectedness with others. Clinicians need to be aware of and sensitive to a family's hierarchy of needs: it is not prudent to address parenting ideas when mom is worried about how she is going to feed her children. The only thing a clinical supervisor ever knew to tell me about working with impoverished communities was that I should not make an appointment before 11:00 a.m. Everything else about working successfully with low-resource families I learned from clients who were themselves socioeconomically challenged.

It was heartbreaking to see families who had fallen between the cracks and were unable to acquire services that were desperately needed to live safely and securely. The stories of two families, challenged to meet their basic needs, are presented next. The Smith family had secured temporary housing while on the waiting list for "Section 8" housing. I accompanied one of our therapists—we'll call him "T"—to their home during a supervisory home visit. They greeted us warmly at the door: mom, dad, and three young children. Each moved toward their usual place to sit, including T, and I looked around. The family pointed toward the open end of the room, inviting me to sit. My choices were either a very old, lumpy, and stained loveseat; or the floor. The floor was covered with old, stringy shag carpeting that was worn, but looked better than the loveseat. I picked a place on the floor in front of the loveseat, facing the family, and sat there.

I found myself thinking about this family's dilemma. Both parents worked full time. Their three young children required childcare. Clearly, they wanted to pay their own way and be independent of social services. During a time when they were having problems with the availability of affordable childcare providers, they had left the children home alone for a few hours, and had been reported to Child Welfare when the kids wandered down the street. Now they had additional burdens and expenses because of a case plan and court hearings. They were on a waiting list for subsidized housing, but no subsidies would be available for childcare because two working parents earning more than $10 or $12 an hour each at that time made too much money to qualify. The child welfare system could afford to provide them a case manager and case manager supervisor, an IFS family therapist, and a public defender; but not the actual resource—childcare—that would have alleviated their core issue and benefited the children.

Child Welfare's assessment found that both parents had grown up in families with parents who were addicted to alcohol and drugs. Mom had been diagnosed with bi-polar during her teenage years and was taking psychotropic medications prescribed by a primary care physician. Dad was a recovering alcoholic. He sought help on his own prior to the Child Welfare intervention and was participating in Alcoholics Anonymous. His disclosure to IFS was that he did not want his drinking to hurt his children the way his parents' addiction had caused harm in his family of origin. Two of his siblings were addicted to drugs, and in and out of hospitals for addiction treatment. His sister had married an alcoholic and was killed when the car her husband was driving swerved into the wrong lane. "I love my children too much to put them through what I've been through," was the father's statement that the Child Protective Services (CPS) investigator had written in her report.

The session with the family was going well and I noted T's skills at facilitating the discussion and eliciting solutions from the family. They obviously liked and trusted him. T was addressing child behavioral issues and mental health concerns that were impacting the family. I provided feedback to the family and was looking at the parents for their response when peripherally I noticed a black furry animal scurry by and disappear. No one reacted to it. The parents had been looking at each other, and the children had been watching for their father's reaction, so I wasn't sure if anyone else had seen it. I thought to myself, "I hope they have a cat." The therapy session continued, and I waited until we got outside to ask T, "The family has a black cat, right?" T responded, "No, the family doesn't have a cat."

Staying Safe in Sketchy Neighborhoods

We worked with the spectrum of social classes, gender identities, cultures and ethnicities, races, disabilities, family dynamics, biases, criminal histories, traumas, and personal tragedies. Clinical staff were able to recognize potentially competent parents under layers of dysfunction, difficult histories, emotional pain, and trauma. Some of our most significant talents involved the ability to gain the trust and cooperation of families and communities who did not have reason to trust by virtue of having been betrayed by the system and professionals for decades or even generations. SFBT, non-blaming and empowering, provided for most families the first positive experience with a clinical approach and therapist. Our after-service follow-up by researchers at three months, six months, and one year confirmed that our efforts and the changes those families made were genuine and continued after discharge.

We prioritized employee safety and were careful to avoid situations that were not safe; although, depending on an individual's life experiences, some of the environments that we would call "quirky" or "uncomfortable" might be regarded by others as untenable. On the rare occasion when in-home therapy was regarded as too risky with a particular family, or under otherwise extraordinary circumstances, approval could be granted for therapy to occur at a neutral site or in our offices. Safety concerns were sometimes obvious—as in the case where a family in a rural, secluded setting had a towering flagpole flying a "Don't tread on me" flag, and a sign on the front door that read, "No Trespassing. Trespassers will be shot. If You are from the Government, You are Trespassing."

Therapists who had never experienced clients living in multigenerational poverty, rural secluded communities, ghettos, or inner-city neighborhoods influenced by gangs initially felt uncomfortable and on high alert. Once we learned how to communicate with residents and neighborhood leaders, staff adjusted to the challenges. Teaming new employees with a seasoned in-home therapist was often helpful. Our clinicians quickly learned the unwritten rules, such as: "Learn the neighborhood standards and be respectful"; "Ask the family where they want you to sit, but whenever possible sit on hard surfaces, not cloth"; and "Bring your own beverages." Families were protective of us and made sure that their neighbors knew we were invited. In fact, with very few exceptions, families loved their therapists—although they might have regarded their case manager, the court, or Child Welfare as adversaries. Bottom line: they made sure we were safe.

Mattie: "I Live for Their Future to be Better than I Ever Could Have Imagined"

"Turf rules" in neighborhoods were communicated among staff. When we needed to provide services for families living in areas dominated by gangs, we were careful and followed the steps necessary to at least achieve safety for ourselves and our families. Mattie—a widowed mother of daughters ages ten and 12—feared for their wellbeing and future. She lived in subsidized housing populated with adult and juvenile gangs. There were occasional shootings, robberies, and assaults in the neighborhood. Mattie worked full time as a senior warehouse records clerk. Her salary after the rent for subsidized public housing was barely adequate to support her and the girls. Mattie's employer regarded her as a dependable and hardworking employee, and Mattie was proud to have held her full-time job for almost nine years.

Mattie grew up under difficult circumstances, yet held traditional family values and a strong work ethic. Both of her parents were drug addicts and incarcerated by the time she was seven years old. Mattie lived in 11 foster homes until she was 18. During the first semester of her senior year, the child welfare agency with legal custody told her to get a job and save money because she was going to be released from their jurisdiction once she graduated. After graduating, Mattie married her teenage boyfriend, the father of her children; but shortly after their fourth wedding anniversary, he died from a cancer that had been in remission for a time. Sadly, he had not been able to secure a bone marrow transplant that might have saved him. Mattie was left straddled with hefty monthly payments for her husband's medical bills and other expenses.

Self-supporting from the time of her husband's death, Mattie had always struggled to make ends meet, yet did not compromise her values, refusing offers to affiliate with a gang and be involved in crimes including thefts and drug sales. "I kept focused on staying clean and setting the right example for my children," she told us. The initial reason Mattie had a case plan under Child Welfare was because a report was made, by the children's school, that she resided in a high-risk drug, prostitution, and criminal gang area; and that due to her working hours, the children were home without childcare or adult supervision for up to two hours some days. Her dilemma was not unusual for single parents of color in that community.

Further inquiries and corroborative reports also alleged that Mattie had a gang-affiliated boyfriend. Mattie was honest when she addressed the allegations. Her explanation to Child Welfare and the court was that she had to work; that private childcare was not affordable and was not offered to her; that public housing had not provided her with other options for apartments; and that it was unsafe for a single mom not to have at least a casual boyfriend from within the "projects" for protection. Mattie's efforts at being placed on waiting lists for subsidized housing elsewhere were not sufficient to prevent a complaint of neglect from being substantiated.

Mattie continued to search for additional family resources, including childcare, without success. Child Welfare placed the children into temporary shelter care and looked for housing and childcare options. As had been Mattie's experience, Child Welfare's attempts to secure alternative housing and affordable childcare for Mattie were fruitless, and the case manager acknowledged Mattie's difficult situation. A case plan meeting was scheduled for two weeks in the future, and the family was assigned to a new protective services unit that worked with parents of children who were in temporary foster care. The meeting did not go smoothly between Mattie and the newly assigned Child Welfare case manager. Mattie was frantic that her children would be victimized by a foster care nightmare like the one she had experienced as a child. The stress overwhelmed her, and she complained of chest pains and exhibited symptoms of depression.

In court, a family resource agency that advocated for single parent families asked the judge not to order the children to remain in foster care, and to instead direct Child Welfare to return the children home, enroll the children into an out-of-district school that had sliding-scale latchkey childcare on site, and refer the family to IFS. The court accepted the recommendation, and an IFS referral meeting was held. It was emphasized that foster placement was imminent if we did not accept this family. Mattie's physical and emotional symptoms were interfering with her functioning, so her ability to continue employment was also at risk. Mattie's risk assessment would have appeared on the lower-priority tier for IFS services; but we accepted Mattie and her daughters as in-home clients, confident that a mental health evaluation would confirm a need for our services. We had no doubt that she was a deserving client, in crisis, and at imminent risk of losing custody of her children.

The public housing apartment where Mattie lived was a "clinic" of gangland occupation and activity. It was a two-story apartment building, with ground-floor and second-floor apartments. Each apartment had an exterior door facing a semicircular open courtyard. A wide, external stairway with iron banisters ran up the center of the building, meeting the second-story elevated walkway that ran from end to end. Mattie's apartment was on the lower level, close to the end on the right side. Two young adult males sat on the center stairs, about one-third of the way up. It was obvious that they were guarding access to the upstairs and acting as lookouts. There could be no doubt that one or more of the upstairs apartments were being used for both prostitution and drug sales. From our car, we had observed several young adults approaching the lookouts, and then being directed to upstairs apartments.

Seasoned IFS therapists were aware of the protocols that governed these situations. For example, it is best not stay after dark; if your vehicle gets "tagged" (i.e., spray painted or otherwise defaced), do not come back; and first secure permission from the family and the neighborhood before beginning in-home therapy. Without these precautions, IFS and the family could both be at risk. We knew to follow the "rules," stay out of the gang's business, and reassess safety issues with each appointment. Our safety protocols included leaving our agency personnel with information about the time and location of each appointment; and checking in regularly.

We approached the two lookouts and before we got too close, said:

> We are not cops; we are counselors. We are here with permission of one of the families to help mom and her daughters. We've been asked to come two or three days a week for a couple of hours; and we mind our own business.

They told us to continue to our appointment after asking which apartment our client lived in. Then one of them said, "You don't want to be here much after dark; and always check in when you get here." They also issued a clear warning that translated as, "Don't cross us."

During our first in-home therapy appointment, we explained to Mattie and her daughters that we would continue with in-home therapy as long as it was safe for us to do so, and we needed to rely on them to share any safety information that might be relevant. We also discussed alternatives to in-home services in order to let them know that we had a backup plan for them; although, as it turned out, we were able to complete services in the family's apartment without interruption. After a couple of weeks, the gang lookouts decided that they liked us. They began to greet us as if we were old friends. Over the years, we had two other families referred from that neighborhood and the lookouts welcomed IFS therapists whenever we approached. Stories about the tough guys, drug sales, and prostitution occurring "next door" became part of the IFS folklore.

Mattie's daughters were excellent students, well-behaved, and insightful about their surroundings and circumstances. Mattie clearly stated from the onset of services:

> My children will complete high school and college. They will become somebody. No foster care homes for them. They know that I love them and will always love them. I live for their future to be better than I could ever have imagined for my life!

Mattie found the time to do homework and study with them, and sometimes tutor them, having to first learn the school curriculum herself. Every Saturday she would take them to the library to do research on whatever interested them, and to read for pleasure. "They are scholarship potential," one of the school counselors told us. "Top of their class—and testing is well above grade level."

Our intervention helped Mattie to address depression and lingering emotional issues from separation, grief, and loss that manifested from losing her parents to drugs; growing up in multiple foster homes; and unresolved grief over her husband's death. Her children gained perspective, self-confidence, and an appreciation for their mother's history and coping skills. They knew they were loved. We acknowledged and built on Mattie's strengths and resilience. Although time-limited with this family, we were able to make referrals and advocate for Mattie to secure housing in a better neighborhood, as well as finding additional resources for the children. This was a rewarding, heartwarming referral for IFS.

Goals and the "Miracle Question"

We learned that when the risk of harm is high, goal setting needs to occur concurrently during the assessment process. Our best practice standards dictated that we elicit goals from the family beginning with the first day of contact. The setting of goals with IFS clients was an integral cornerstone of the collaborative therapeutic alliance. Where a family has "everything" to lose, goals contribute greatly to creating hope, willingness, and confidence; reducing risk; strengthening the therapeutic alliance; promoting a customer relationship for therapy; and getting off to a fast start. Goals also are helpful in focusing a client's attention on acknowledging and addressing the issues or problems around the reasons for referral.

Goals that are elicited from clients can provide both direction in therapy and benchmarks for therapists and clients to document progress. Goals should be realistic and broken down into small increments achievable in less than three weeks. Well-defined, workable goals elicited from clients in the client's own words are goals that are owned by the client. Those goals should be in the client's control; concrete, specific and in behavioral terms; and perceived by the client as requiring effort. Additionally, goals should be expressed in affirmative language. For example, "sobriety" with increments or steps elicited from the client is better than "not drinking" as a goal. Stating a goal as "communicating calmly in a non-blaming way" with descriptions of what that looks like, elicited from the client, will work better than "not arguing" as a goal (O'Hanlon & Weiner-Davis 1989, pp. 101-102). In every case, we need to ask:

- "When have you already done that, at least a little bit, in the past?"
- "How did you do that?"
- "What needs to happen for you to do more of it?"

"A powerful way of helping people to focus on potential solutions rather than on problems is the miracle question" (Cade and O'Hanlon 1993, p. 101). The "miracle question" was the premier goal-setting question for IFS. It works well with individuals, couples, and families. In addition to identifying concrete goals and layers of goals that clients desire, the miracle question helps to set a foundation for future fast-forward and scaling questions, incremental change benchmarks, and ideas for tasks. IFS family therapists processed the miracle question with the whole family; and each member had the opportunity to identify and detail specifically what their miracle would encompass.

We found that the most productive wording of the miracle question is as follows:

> Do you mind if I ask you a sort of silly question? You go to sleep tonight and while you are sleeping, a miracle happens. All your problems are gone. You don't exactly know yet that your problems are gone when you awake, but you begin to find out through the day, week, and month.

For processing with a family, ask, "Who will notice first that something is different?" Then proceed with a sequence of questions:

- "What's the first thing that you will notice is different?"
- "What will be different at home throughout the day?"
- "What will be different at work/school? At...?"

Write down what the client/family says, in the words of each client.

In a few rare instances, clients expressed some discomfort with the idea of a miracle, so the question was asked again in a modified way: "... *something happens* ..." Our research consultants concluded that the discomfort may have sometimes occurred when newer IFS therapists, who themselves were less than comfortable about asking the miracle question, telegraphed their discomfort to a client without consciously realizing it. The idea of the miracle question is simply to get a client to talk about their life without problems, so there is a video description with words about how things will be for the family when current problems no longer exist.

My personal experience is that clients—especially couples and families with children—really enjoy the participatory process of answering the question and hearing how their partner, parents, siblings, and children envision life absent any current obstacles. Parents and children contribute and build on each other's wishes. As they express how the miracle will look, their emotions resemble what you might see with gift giving. There are smiles, bright eyes, and sometimes even laughter. I could see my clients begin to visualize how things could become better for themselves and their family.

Follow-up questions continue, and each answer becomes a goal that is reflective of how the client wants their life and relationships to be. The goals—which are realistic and in the client's control—become actual measurable goals that we can process, document, and follow. If some answers are not in the client's control—for example, "My miracle would be that I would win the lottery"—we can process them in a more realistic fashion by responding, "Oh, so more money would help—what would you do with more money?"

Examples of possible follow up-questions include the following:

- "What will you be noticing? And you? And you?"
- "And what exactly will you be seeing and hearing?"
- "What will be different for you?"
- "Then what will happen?"
- "What will happen next?"
- "Who will be doing/saying what?"
- "What will be different between the two of you?/For you?/And for you?"

The questioning continues to identify some goals throughout the day or over several days. I like to ask:

- "Who else will notice?"
- "What else will then change and be different?"
- "If I were to come to your house and this miracle had just happened, what would I notice that would tell me it had happened?"
- "And then what will happen next?"

I want to be sure that the family talks about changes at home, work, school, and in the family. They can even include family members not in the session. The idea is to create questions to customize this process for your client-family.

When clients are asked at the beginning of future clincial sessions, "What's better?" often parts of their "miracle" will be in their answer; but usually they will not immediately realize it. When that happens, throw success in your client's face by saying something like: "That sounds like part of your miracle. You said that would happen. How did you do that? Tell me more. What else happened? What will be happening next?"

Tasks

Our researchers documented the power of tasking families to promote between session change. To our surprise, we found that even tasks that are vague and unrelated to the problem can be powerful initiators of change. Several of our therapists experienced good outcomes with vague, accidental tasks. One of the stories I've told in my workshops, which speaks to the power of tasking, is about a therapist we will call Jack. Jack was uncomfortable about assigning tasks to a family. He was a fine clinician, but did not have experience or training in tasking strategies. In fact, he thought of tasks as unnecessary at best and manipulative at worst.

When our researchers requested that families be assigned tasks so that the outcomes could be documented, Jack told me that he dreaded ever having to assign a task to one of his client families. I told him that he needed to assign a task to the next family he visited, for our research. Jack asked me, "How should I do it?" My response was:

> Jack, near the end of the appointment, talk with them about a home-work assignment that you think would be helpful to accomplish a goal or interrupt a pattern. Maybe assign them something that they already said they wanted to do.

Jack thought for a minute and responded:

> That makes no sense to me. I still don't get it. What if I give the wrong task? How will I know? What if they don't do it? It seems to me that this will be a minefield for me and my families.

Jack was still unsure about what task to give to the family as he was facilitating the session that evening. Standing by the door at the end of the session and feeling desperate, he told the Jones family that he needed to give them a homework assignment. They assured him that they would do whatever he needed and asked, "Jack, what do we need to do?" Jack frantically looked around and noticed a small table adjacent to their living room. The table had many candles on it; some were partially burned, while others had never been lit. He told them to pick a time when they were all home, stand near the table, and then each select and light their own candle. Mrs. Jones said, "Okay Jack, we can do that. Then what?" Jack thought for a few seconds and then replied, "Well, just stand there for about 20 minutes." Dad asked, "And then?" Jack replied, "You'll know; just do it, please, and we'll talk about it during our next meeting."

Jack described the Jones family as consisting of mom and dad, and two young adolescent girls:

> They've had their share of problems. The kids have been acting out and the parents are busy and preoccupied—too busy for the time the girls need from their parents. We've worked some on communication and time management, but there is a lot of avoidance and either the girls or the parents give up easily and lose patience. Mom can have a temper and dad feels unappreciated. The girls say that they just want to be left alone but they crave time and attention from their parents. The good news is that the girls seem to be invested in our family sessions; but then

again, they often complain about their parents, their life, and school. You know, they're young teens.

The following week, after his next appointment with the family, Jack gleefully strolled into my office with a broad smile on his face. "It worked!" he said, "The task worked!" I replied, "Tell me about it." Jack said he had been met at the door with mom wagging her finger at him, saying, "We know what you were thinking; we know what you were doing." Jack was caught off guard. "What? What?" he responded, not understanding what they were referring to. "You know—the homework," mom reminded him. The family told him they had gathered around the table Sunday night, and each had selected and lit one of the candles, just as Jack had asked. They began to discuss what the purpose of this assignment might be as they watched the candles burn.

Mom explained to Jack:

> And then we got it. Each of us at the same time understood what you were trying to tell us. The candles were like our life together as a family. The candles were getting shorter, just as our time together was getting shorter. We need to be more serious about being close and communicating … About loving each other and listening. Before we know it, the kids will have different lives, and we'll be old, regretting all the things we could have done as parents when the girls were young.

Dad then added, "We're all ready to commit to working on things. There are enough regrets to go around. No more." The family had made something constructive and relevant out of a random task.

At IFS, we learned from our experiences that even though there are several categories of tasks and there may be some merit in strategically developing tasks, the task itself is not as important as what the family does with it. Changing a pattern of behavior or experimenting with how change would look is fundamental to tasking. And when a family modifies a task or does a task differently than assigned, it is constructive more often than not. We found it was very effective to take a short break near the end of the session and then use about the last ten minutes to give the clients positive feedback and praise; talk about their strengths and opportunities; and then discuss a task that would help them complete one segment or increment of what they said they wanted to accomplish. Our outcomes supported the idea that asking clients to do what they say they want is highly efficacious.

It is important not to directly ask families if they have done the task, but instead to wait for them to bring it up—hopefully while answering the "What's better?" question. If they do not initially bring up anything about doing the task, later in the session I sometimes ask, "What part of the task did you do?" because sometimes families modify tasks to fit what they need. And I like to think that if they say that they have not done the task, it is because it was not a task in which they were invested; so I might ask them, "What did you do instead?" The purpose of the task is not to make the therapist feel brilliant, but rather for the family to change a pattern, complete part of a goal, or experiment by doing something different. Most important is for positive change to occur; it does not matter if it comes out of a specific task or just arbitrarily.

IFS Clinicians

IFS clinicians were a hodgepodge of highly skilled and dedicated professionals from all regions of the United States, Canada, and Puerto Rico, who were recruited through professional journals, employment ads, and referrals from other therapists. Screenings and interviews emphasized a strong academic background plus experience and proven success with complex multicultural families. Therapists were expected "on the fly" to accept a different way of thinking about change and become proficient in new clinical strategies and methods driven by research. They were also asked to embrace in-home family therapy in urban, suburban, rural, or very rural areas.

Highly regarded, experienced urban therapists, who had thrived working in private practice primarily with middle-class families, had to make significant adjustments. Not all our hires were able to get beyond the challenges during the first three months; and the rate of pay—although adequate—was not nearly equivalent to the long hours, risks, and complexities of the job. We could not retain about one-third of our newly hired clinicians for even six months because of the complexities of learning the model and the intensity of the issues. Those who embraced the work stayed with us for years, and loved supplementing their clinical toolbox with the research and successes resulting from powerful interventions that benefited a challenging population who desperately needed help.

So why would a successful, licensed therapist work in these environments when private practice or outpatient agencies offered a "cleaner" alternative, a less intense clientele, plus a higher average rate of pay? A psychiatrist who sometimes consulted for us when children were on medication shared his perspective, using medical specialties as a metaphor:

> Some medical doctors select specialties that are more apt to avoid blood, trauma, and death. Ophthalmology is a clean choice and pays higher than most medical specialties. Why would someone choose emergency medicine or become a trauma surgeon when ophthalmology offers a set schedule with few emergencies, mostly office work, some of the highest rates of pay for procedures, and relatively clean work?

He continued:

> like emergency room doctors or trauma surgeons, it's as if you at IFS are constantly on the verge of a code blue. You never know what you will face at work on any given day; and I'd bet the income is not nearly the highest among the psychotherapy specialties.

Traditional Methods Produce Marginal Results

Some of our new clinicians, who were "married to" traditional interventions, were slower to envision the potential for strong outcomes afforded by client-need-driven solution therapies. Others were "sold" almost from the start. One of the highly skilled, open-minded but traditional therapists who observed three family sessions with me shortly after her hire remarked about SFBT: "It's like magic!" She, like many others, became motivated to learn and apply new methods that helped improve outcomes for families while reducing risks to children and society. Accidental discoveries—"I just happened to assign that task" or "I just pulled that one out of the air"— inspired new interventions that were tested, studied, and often adopted as standard practice. We knew that what we were doing was important even beyond the immediate benefit to the client-families with whom we interacted.

IFS client-families—whether struggling with poverty and social injustices, or financially comfortable and enjoying some advantages of social privilege—faced challenges that were difficult, and their case outcome stories would be considered heroic and inspiring by any measure. Our services were family centered and flexible, tailored to accommodate the needs of each family. Families came to love us; and the success of IFS with Child Welfare clients made a marked impression on administrators and legislators. Our initial two years of preserving high-risk families resulted in the allocation of state and county monies to expand IFS programming and research for as much as an additional eight years. The legislature was probably motivated not so much by altruistic factors as by the reduction in tax dollars needed to support children in therapeutic foster care.

During the last few years of the IFS clinical study, several child welfare agencies were subject to consent decrees as a result of lawsuits filed in many states. The court monitors and trainers were very complimentary when they evaluated IFS programming and borrowed IFS strength-based and solution practices as core recommendations for all of Child Welfare. After the IFS research project concluded, I was offered the opportunity to be an independent contractor providing child and family team meeting, culture and diversity, family-centered practice, and solution-oriented brief therapy (B SOFT) training for Child Welfare staff in several jurisdictions and states. B SOFT is SFBT with the addendums from IFS research.

All workshops featured an additional day for roleplay and practice. Some workshops included live demonstration sessions with families referred by case manager attendees. Written reference guides on neurolinguistics, question sequences, goal-setting ideas, tasking, and therapeutic process were included for participants. The hope was that if the CPS, ongoing Child Welfare, and community Mental Health staff would employ some of the intervention ideas that worked for IFS, families would thrive and there would be better outcomes among the Child Welfare population.

See also Appendix H for a peek into the culture and challenges—some self-inflicted—of child welfare agencies.

References

Berg, I. K., and Kelly, S. (2000). *Building Solutions in Child Protective Services*. New York: Norton.

Cade, B., and O'Hanlon, W. (1993). *A Brief Guide to Brief Therapy*. New York: Norton.

Gypen, L., Vanderfaeillie, J., De Maeyer, S., Belenger, L., and Van Holen, F. (2017). Outcomes of children who grew up in foster care: *Systematic Children and Youth Services Review*, Vol. 76. May 2017, pp. 74–83.

Hannan, M., Martin, K., Carceres, K., and Aledort, N. (2017). *Children at Risk: Foster Care and Human Trafficking*. Cham: Springer International.

O'Hanlon, W., and Weiner-Davis, M. (1989). *In Search of Solutions*. New York: Norton, pp. 101–102.

Shirk, M., and Stangler, G. (2004). *On Their Own: What Happens to Kids who Age Out in Foster Care*. Cambridge, MA: Perseus Books.

12 Marriage and Couples Work
A Higher Responsibility

Several decades ago, I attended a workshop on confidentiality and ethics that was facilitated by an attorney. He informed us that, statutorily, marriage is granted special privilege and is given a "higher protected status." The content of his workshop fit with my training as a marriage and family therapist to preserve the marriage and family whenever possible—of course, with consideration to personal safety issues. Ironically, his comments were partially in answer to a question that had been asked during a discussion about the ethical prohibitions forbidding a therapist from engaging in a sexual relationship with a client. The attorney said if he were to defend a clinician who had been caught in a romantic relationship with a client, he would advise the couple to marry immediately. The attorney explained that the legal protections around marriage are so sacred that he believed the state and licensing board would be unable to successfully impose ethical or legal consequences on the therapist he was defending.

I do not know for certain if he is correct about the legal outcome of such a scenario, but I have verified that he is correct about marriage having a protected legal status. As therapists, we have a responsibility to preserve marriage and the family whenever possible, if it is the goal of the client. Family therapists must remain neutral toward partners and honor the relationship, not the individual, as the client. Spouses or partners need to agree that in couples therapy, there is no confidentiality or privacy between them. Clinical records are the joint property of the couple, so any release of documents would require both signatures. I would advocate that neither could attend individual counseling with their couples therapist; in order to remain neutral and honor the relationship, a therapist cannot hold secrets or ethically maintain confidentiality with one of the partners outside of the couples sessions.

DOI: 10.4324/9781003397380-12

Giggles, Exceptions, and Couples Tasking

I attended a couples counseling workshop in the 1990s that was both entertaining and informative. The trainer told the group that he had a foolproof task that could be given to help couples whose complaint was that they "argue all of the time." He presented it this way: after you listen to the couple talk about how they argue all the time, tell them that you have a solution for them, but you don't want to tell them about it unless they first agree that they will do it. (This is called a "devil's deal." The idea is to get a client to agree to do something before you even tell them what you are asking them to do.) Once they agree, you tell them: "At the very first sign that a disagreement is beginning, you are both to get naked—take everything off. Only then, after you both are naked, can you resume your argument." Of course, the whole room erupted in laughter.

His point is that most couples—maybe all couples—cannot argue when they are naked, perhaps because they feel vulnerable or are uncomfortable in another way. When we are naked and beginning to argue, our first impulse is to pull the covers over ourselves or get dressed. The idea behind this task is that at least one of four things are likely to happen: either the couple will get naked and stop the argument; or the couple will be distracted and argue instead about getting naked, as one will start to take clothes off and insist that the other get naked as well; or the couple will think about the task and begin to laugh, or at least be distracted from arguing; or the argument will continue but half-heartedly because they are thinking that they should take their clothes off. Regardless, the pattern of arguing will be interrupted; and the distraction will often create a pause. He believed that the pause would increase awareness and reason, while perhaps reducing the seriousness of the moment. Was he correct?

When I tell this story in my workshops, participants laugh. Workshop attendees hope to be entertained, which is not the hope or expectation of a couple in therapy. When couples enter therapy, they are often stressed out, anxious, even embarrassed. Usually, one if not both partners will present as a complainant. I would advocate for the completion of a thorough intake with a history for each partner, including a cultural history, followed by a relationship history. There are informed consents to sign, including one cautioning them that when couples bring issues to therapy, there is a risk that the relationship can get worse. Sometimes couples will cooperate at intake, which in itself could be an "exception" to refer to in a later session. If there is chronic arguing, I try to gauge the frequency and intensity, and learn what I can about the subject matter. Most often, couples have tried a number of things to resolve their differences or conflicts before opting for therapy. It is a vulnerable time, so any task needs to be a custom fit for the couple's situation and the positions (visitor, complainant, customer) of each individual.

It is true that most couples laugh when they hear the "get naked" story, and it will probably lighten the mood in the room. Even so, I might hold off telling a couple the "get naked" story. The risk is that they will regard it as a tool to use—essentially as an implied task. I need to be relatively certain that any story or task I introduce will be helpful to their relationship, and will not diminish their hope or commitment to therapy. When I know that each partner is truly invested in the relationship and has shown the will and determination to make changes, I can be more confident that creative tasks—even "silly stuff" to change patterns and introduce fun—will be helpful and not do harm. It helps greatly if they are customers over completing a "do something different" task. If a "silly" task to interrupt a pattern is introduced, the couple must be open and willing to try something "outside the box," even absurd. It can be disarming, and maybe tension reducing, when a "silly task" is presented in a manner that is nonchalant and off-the-cuff.

Keep in mind that there is a strategy in solution work that involves the introduction of an "implied task" in lieu of a more direct presentation. There are times when our clinical judgment might tell us not to give a client direct feedback or a task—perhaps because that client may take it as criticism or be uncomfortable for some other reason. We can instead use metaphor or tell a story and see what the client ultimately does with it. Knowing some of the intricacies that can affect our client and their relationships with others can be invaluable in determining how to address some of the more sensitive issues when we ask about exceptions or give feedback and compliments. When working with a couple, sometimes understanding the "backstory" can be important to determine any precipitating factors that could impact differences in the motivation and agenda of each partner. Secrets between partners, or even between the couple and the therapist, can exist and complicate what otherwise might be a direct, clearly indicated intervention.

Traditional methods for reducing a couple's conflict and arguing have included work on communication. My marriage and family therapy licensure internship included practice with a "wand" that was passed back and forth between the partners. The rule was that you could only speak when you were holding the wand. Speaking meant you expressed feelings with "I ..." statements and did not begin a sentence with "You ..." The partner not holding the wand was expected to be a great listener and not think about responses, especially defensive responses. Instead, when the partner with the wand had finished making their point, the other partner was expected to give feedback that demonstrated understanding— for example, "I hear you. You are saying that you were hurt when ... and you are asking me to not do that again." This practice did introduce some skills in communication, including listening skills; but I have never been confident that it carried over to the moment when the couple was on the verge of blowing up!

Solution strategies set the table for an effective outcome. Naturally, at intake and during the first several sessions that follow, there is time for "problem talk," so that the couple can provide a vivid picture of their issues and concerns, and I have a chance to listen and reflect back an understanding of their presenting problem. But problem talk is only one piece of the intake process. At some point early in the process, I will likely ask: "What are the things in your life that you are happy about and don't want to change?" Several sessions into our work, if the couple is not in immediate crisis, our meetings will begin with the question: "What's better?" It is not unusual for couples, between sessions when they are anticipating that the "What's better?" question will be asked, to look for or perhaps create a situation that is "better."

When the general problem is, "We don't have fun anymore—the marriage is the problem," after acknowledging their frustration, I might challenge that premise with, "There must have been a time last week when things were better—a day or a few hours when things went well; maybe a day that was just a little bit better?" When I hear an answer that illustrates an exception to their problem, I engage them in a discussion of details and then follow up with a process that includes questions such as the following:

- "How did you do that?
- "Who initiated it?"
- "Then what happened?
- "What did you do; and what did [the other] do?"
- "How did you know to do that?"
- "What needs to happen for you to do more of that?"

Their answers usually provide clues to some of the strengths in their relationship, what they want to do more of, and a task that might be productive.

Couples in crisis who complain about arguing all the time can pose additional challenges, especially if there are old issues or a legacy of betrayals. I need to hear about the history of those deeper problems and what the couple has already done to try to resolve them. Acknowledging their strengths and commitment, and then complimenting them on their efforts to work things out, usually goes a long way to motivate them and build hope. Then I can pursue "exceptions" to the arguing: "You said that you argue all the time; but there must have been a time last week—maybe a day or hour—when you got along and didn't argue. What day or part of a day was that?" Once they come up with a day or time, I pursue with them what was good about that day; what was different; how they did it; what needs to happen for them to have more days like that one, etc. After a session or two, I might even have them remember a time when they began to argue but stopped and because of that, things worked out well. "How did you know to stop at that moment?"

Listening to problems, giving feedback for understanding and hope, and asking for exceptions will create a strong foundation on which to build. It is important to then give compliments, emphasize the strengths of each partner and the couple, and point out how each has contributed to making things work better. When I point out strengths, I might tell the couple, "It's easy to lose sight of your strengths along the way, but you can fix that." Likely, there is a task that I can give to the couple based on what they said they have already done that worked, or perhaps what they said they wanted to do more of:

> You said that both of you enjoyed going to the movies and dinner Wednesday night, and what made it especially good for you [wife] is that your husband planned it. I heard you say that you wanted to have more evenings like that, and you wouldn't mind planning some yourself. So, who will be planning the next date night that will include surprises, and what night will it be?

I am thrilled to be the "excuse" they use for enjoying time together; or having a meaningful discussion; or making the effort to overcome a conflict with a risky, difficult conversation. Let them say, "We did it because our therapist told us that we needed to do it." No matter. When they do it and it works, they are accomplishing at least one of their goals. They deserve the credit for initiating it and following through. The therapist is merely the catalyst!

Couples therapy can be very involved and tricky. Completing classes in the fundamentals and attending exceptional "hands-on" workshops provided by highly regarded clinicians have been helpful; although what I have learned in vivo directly from client couples has been most valuable. Couples often have everything they need to solve their problems, and even can have fun doing it. If this idea sounds like Milton Erickson's thinking, it is because it is similar! Erickson believed and demonstrated in his work that clients usually have everything they need to resolve their issues and build the happiness they desire. I first heard about this concept from clinicians who were familiar with Erickson's work and writings; but then I learned it from my clients.

Ann and Tom: "If Only We Could Go Back"

As with any modality, I have learned that the blueprint for intervention involves listening to what the couple tells me, understanding each partner's philosophy of change, and hearing exceptions and solutions. Ann and Tom, distressed by a relationship that had become "boring, mundane, and wrought with conflict," had provided me with information I needed to help them put their solutions into action.

Ann and Tom presented as anxious, nervous, and emotionally stressed. Forty-eight-year-old Ann and 50-year-old Tom were asking for marriage counseling "as a last resort," reporting that they had been unhappy for at least the last ten years of their 24-year marriage. They met while attending college, lived together for four years, and then got married. They described themselves as "empty nesters," although they emphasized that their two daughters leaving home—one a senior in college and the other now graduated and self-supporting—did not contribute to their unhappiness.

Ann characterized their relationship during the past 12 years as awful, unhappy, and in a boring routine. Tom agreed with her, explaining that the romance had died many years ago, and each of them had then had to find new friends, activities, and interests independent of the other. Tom said that they had stayed together for the kids only, and he had been grieving the loss of their previously romantic, exciting, and fun relationship of more than ten years. Ann nodded as Tom discussed his sadness and their history of attempts over the years to "reignite the spark and laughter." Vacations together, "date nights," road trips with the kids that included couple's time away from the kids, attending plays and comedy acts, and nostalgic visits to their hometowns did not help to reinvigorate their relationship.

Both Ann and Tom were strong believers in personal responsibility and prided themselves on their successful parenting, which included passing on values of responsibility and charity to their daughters. They supported a local organization with donations of money and their personal time, believing that a helping hand can make a difference for almost anyone. They told me that the message they wanted to bring to disadvantaged and disenfranchised families is: "We can help a little bit; but you need to do the rest for yourself." They were proud of their charity work and support for the community charity that promoted a philosophy of "personal responsibility" consistent with theirs.

Ann worked as a business manager for a regional medical center and Tom was a high-school teacher. They recalled struggling financially during the first several years of marriage, dreaming of a time when they would be settled in their careers and have enough money not to worry. Now that they were financially secure, they said it was ironic that they longed for those days when they were uncertain about having a sufficient paycheck.

During the intake session, Ann said, "I don't believe we'll make it to our silver anniversary"; while Tom replied, with sarcasm in his voice, "We know how to suffer together." I noted that although they said that they were challenged to find new friends, activities, and interests together, they had mentioned the charity work as something that they did together. I remarked that there must be other things and asked them what they did well together. They each talked about their mutual hobby of almost 20 years: performing as amateur actors at the community center theatre. Ann's description of their hobby was:

> We are really good at acting and do two or three plays a year. We love it—it's something we're both good at, and we complement each other when we play opposite as hero and heroine or villain. I think we sort of compete to be the "better actor," and maybe that makes each of us better. Acting is my number one joy these days. Even work has become too routine and there are no options for me to advance or leave.

Ann paused tearfully and added, as she began to cry, "But now at home our life is too serious. We've raised our kids, gotten older, and I guess I forgot how to have fun." Tom added, "If only we could go back—back to when things were enjoyable, when anyone could see we were in love. It's that same old story: 'If only I knew then what I know now.' But you can't go back." I could hear the sadness in their voices. Processing feelings of grief and loss over their relationship would be contraindicated. They needed a way to move forward and find happiness again; and they needed to have some fun!

They had given me their task and part of a potential solution without realizing it. I complimented them on their insights, and the efforts they made over the years to stay together:

> I know your children really benefited from your commitment to stay together during their growing years. Plus, the values you've given to them are life changers that will always benefit them. They are thriving because of you. Your parenting is a tribute to the love you have for them.

I continued the conversation with compliments until I could see that they had leveled out emotionally. Then I told them:

> I can help you, but it's going to take hard work on your part. I will be asking you at the critical time if you're ready, truly ready, to work to turn things around; but first I need some information so I can understand your relationship better.

Ann and Tom looked at me curiously and each committed to do whatever was needed if it was truly possible to make things better. I said:

> This is really important. There are things that I need to understand about each of you and your relationship. I am asking you to tell me about a time when you were happy and in love, could converse with one another, and would have told me that you were in a wonderful, caring, and loving relationship. When would that have been?

After a short back and forth, they agreed on a time during the first five years of their cohabitating/early marriage. I then asked them to describe in detail what a day, and then what a week, would have been like during that time. As they talked about things they would have said and done, I asked for more and more detail while giving them feedback that reflected on how loving things must have been for them during that time. Their descriptions began to sound more enthusiastic, and their moods lightened—even evolving into laughter at times—as they recalled some of their trials and tribulations back at a time when they were somewhat naïve about the world.

I gave them a simple task as the session ended:

> Let's get together five days from now, next Tuesday. Between now and then, I want you to talk more about that year when things were great, and you were a happy couple. Please write down whatever you remember and bring it to our next meeting. I need all the information you can provide with enough detail to give me a clear and accurate picture. Then I will be able to help you.

I asked them specifically what days they would be able to work on the list and had them commit to putting time aside on those days. Then I scaled them from 0-10 both on their willingness to follow through with the assignment and on their confidence to do it. From my years involved in research, I've learned that unless clients are a 9 or 10 on both scales, they likely will not do the task. If a client is less than a 9, I ask them how the task can be modified to make it a 9 or 10. Each of them said they were a 10 on both the willingness and confidence scales, so I did not need to modify the task.

During the first part of the next session, when I asked them the "What's better?" question, Ann and Tom referred to their list and reported that it has been fun for them to relive some of the memories from their early years together. I laughed with them, and observed how great things must have been during those years. At times, during their disclosure, I would ask,

"How did you do that? How did you get through that? How did you stay hopeful and upbeat?" as they brought up times when they had struggled to find work; decide on where to live; grieve Tom's mother's death; and pay rent or buy groceries when one or both were between jobs. They were able to recall how they had problem solved together and remained hopeful even in challenging times; but I could see an underlying sadness. I surmised that they were missing the way their relationship had been, and some of those memories might be provoking feelings of yearning for what they once had. I processed their "mixed" feelings during a pause in their disclosure.

Near the end of the session, they asked me what my idea was to help them. I told them:

> Actually, it was more of your idea than mine. If you are willing to commit to seriously considering an experiment that may require a sustained effort, and some of your acting skills and talents, we can talk about it. Before I tell you what the assignment is, I need to be sure that you are serious about making your marriage work.

They both affirmed that they were, and then I told them: "This will require both of you to work together; to be serious about doing this, but to also have fun with it. I guess we'll find out if you are truly great actors." Ann and Tom indicated that now they were really eager to hear my idea. I explained:

> I am asking you to pretend one day next week—just for one day, and no more than one day—that it is 15 or 20 years ago, and you are truly in love and having fun. Make it real. Say things and do things that would be consistent with being in love; having a true couple alliance; being calm, light, and upbeat; going out and having fun. Reenact the feelings and mood of your relationship 15 or 20 years ago.

They posed a few questions about the parts they would be playing and asked for some instructions and guidelines. My reply was that it was totally up to them, and they would have to invent things on the fly: "I would think you've had some experience with adlibbing."

Jay Haley (1987) and Cloé Madanes (1981) have used what they call "pretend directives" in interventions with clients, including for couples seeking help. As strategic therapists, their interventions will typically focus on the problems and the problems as symptoms. "Directives" are used to modify or reduce the power of the problems. Solution therapists do not direct clients. Interventions are collaborative; and what are called "tasks" or "homework" generally reflect doing all or part of the solution— in other words, what the client says they want. In SFBT, there are four possibilities: the client will do the task; do part of the task; not do the task; or do something different. If a client does not do the task, the assumption is that it was the wrong task, and the clinician apologizes for having erred or missed something. In strategic therapy, there is another option reflective of the "clinician is the expert philosophy": "With a not-so-nice-response, the therapist should have the attitude that the family has failed ... they have failed themselves. The therapist condemns them for unfortunately having missed an opportunity" (Haley 1987. pp. 71-72).

I asked the couple, "What day would work for you both?" They looked at their schedules and both agreed on Saturday. I continued:

Okay, so you might want to rehearse things in your minds between now and then and make plans. Maybe you will want to gather some props or put plans in place before then. But wait for Saturday to go full bore; although it would be okay to just practice informally a little before Saturday. Just remember, no matter what: you're on stage Saturday, as if you're in front of an audience—maybe even critics.

They smiled from time to time as we talked, then agreed to the task, scaling their willingness and confidence at 10. For the balance of the session, they maintained eye contact with each other, nodding from time to time. I could see that they were processing ideas about the teamwork and "acting" this would require.

When the couple returned the following week, they were bubbly and laughing in the waiting room. I delayed slightly before inviting them into my office because they sounded like they were having fun and enjoying each other's company. When I asked them, "What's better?" the floodgates opened, and I heard a detailed description of Saturday's experience. I laughed with them and toward the end of the session I said, "You guys are great actors!" Ann smiled and said, "It was easy, and I don't think we were acting most of the day. It became real." Tom nodded. I responded, "You guys are great. I think I hear you—maybe it wasn't only about being great actors; maybe at least some of the time it was about being a great couple." They both smiled. Then they confessed that even though they promised to pretend for just one day, "maybe we carried it on for a longer time—maybe two or three days." They began to tell a story about going out to dinner Sunday night to celebrate how great Saturday had been for them. "We even shared dessert together, like we used to when we didn't have a lot of money."

Tom asked, "So what do we do next?" I paused for a minute and said:

Are you guys talented enough to either be a great couple or act like a great couple for at least two days next week? I was going to say only two, but it sounds like you're not good at following instructions.

They had a contagious laugh, and my poker face became a laughing face. My thinking was, "If it works, do more of it." I have no apprehension in assigning the same task if it works well.

Tom and Ann returned a week later, again touting their success and happiness. The imagined became real for them. Of course, as I had provoked them to do, they disregarded my "for two days" guidance and had a great week together. Knowing that they could make their relationship whatever they wanted it to be was empowering for them: "We had just forgotten how to enjoy each other's company; how to have fun together." What they had done was to model how a "pretend task" can work when it is customized to a client's strengths, goals, and abilities. It did not feel like something strange or unnatural for them to do, and the payoff was everything and more that they had hoped for out of therapy.

My work with this couple was not so much about the therapy as it was about their willingness to get in touch with their strengths as a couple and break a pattern of despair. What they needed was to once again do some of the things that had worked for them in the past. Coming to therapy was a clear message to me that they really wanted their relationship to work. Tying the task to their strengths as actors and their "just do it" personal responsibility values fit well for them. I included in my notes at discharge that Tom's idea, "You can't go back," was incomplete. In the last session, he modified it when he added, "But you can move forward." I have continued to use "pretend tasks" with couples, and more times than not, couples have been able to get in touch with relationship strengths that they had forgotten, and then find ways to create new strengths and solutions.

Runaway Beth, Mom, and Stepdad

It is not unusual for a family to come to therapy with a specific agenda. Clients might ask for family therapy, or perhaps therapy to address a child's behavior, and end up in couples counseling. It is a therapist's job to determine the difference between the "symptom" and the "problem," while attending to the family's agenda. A sure way to lose a client in the beginning of therapy is to tell a parent that they need couples counseling when they have told you the problem is a child's behavior. There are strategies that allow us to respect a client's agenda while helping the family to find the best treatment path. Beth's family is an example of what can work well when the child is the "identified patient," but the marital issues are the precipitating cause.

Arnold and Karen asked the Juvenile Court for help with their daughter, Beth, and they were given a list of clinical providers. They then checked with their insurance company and found me listed as an approved therapist, so they called for an appointment. Karen's 16-year-old daughter, Beth, had run away from home 15 times over three years. Karen had given birth to Beth as a teenager, and Beth never knew her biological father. The circumstances around Karen's pregnancy and Beth's father were described in juvenile justice documents as either unknown or undisclosed. Karen worked to support herself and Beth until Beth finished first grade. The summer before Beth turned seven, Karen married Arnold. They had three children together: Sam, seven, Allison, six, and Katy, four. Karen was able to be a "stay-at-home-mom" because Arnold made an excellent salary; but it required him to work long hours—generally, he left for work before 7:00 a.m. and did not return home until 7:00 p.m. or later.

Arnold and Karen brought Beth to my office, and I took a family history. Beth had always been an A and B student, and was well spoken, sweetly sensitive and clearly insightful. Other than the running away, she had no blemishes on her record. It was clear that she was mature for her age, and an independent thinker. She shrugged and described her runaway episodes as, "It's what I had to do … No big deal—I didn't hurt anyone and I'm old enough to decide things for myself." I asked Beth how she had managed to run away 15 times in such a brief period, and her mother answered for her: "Beth never stays away more than a few weeks."

Karen cried during much of our meeting and did not challenge anything that was said, but made it clear that she was concerned for Beth and loved her husband and children. Arnold had a singular stated agenda: "Beth needs to be obedient and stop running away." He complained that she was out of control and did not respect him as her father. Twice he made the point, "I am the only father she has ever had." Karen and Arnold were expecting me to acknowledge that Beth was the problem and focus on correcting her behavior. I told them that I needed to see them and Beth together for at least one more meeting. Arnold was surprised and said, "Wait—this is serious. I hope you understand. Beth is ruining our marriage and she is probably messing up our kids. She may not mean to do harm, but she is taking down this family."

One concern I had was that the family dynamics resembled a situation where a child—often a stepchild—was being sexually abused. During the family intake, I asked about any abuse including sexual abuse, but I did not have an opportunity to meet alone with Beth. The informed consent allowed me to contact the Juvenile Court and previous therapists. I talked with the Juvenile Court family coordinator and a previous therapist of Beth's, and both assured me that they had explored that possibility and ruled it out. The Family Court coordinator told me that the Juvenile Court had in fact investigated the possibility of abuse, and there was a report I could read. After I reviewed their notes, the report, and details of the investigation from the year before, I also ruled out that possibility.

Beth's stepfather, Arnold, was well meaning; and I think too often there is a tendency among clinicians to take sides with the most vulnerable and give less focus to the agenda of the most dominant or powerful family member. It would be too easy to think, "Poor Beth—something must be going on with her that is just awful. And poor mom—look at what she must be going through, being caught between her husband, her daughter, and the other children." The fact is that everyone in this situation is a good person, well-meaning and wanting to address issues for the sake of the family. Perceptions may be different, but motives are primarily to make things better. So, we need to focus on the family as the client, and keep in mind that working toward making things better for everyone is our responsibility.

I needed a strategy to quickly figure out the family dynamics and understand more about Beth "running away without any reason." I might only have one more session with them! From Arnold's reaction, it did not seem that we had time to go through processing with questions such as, "When did you feel like running away but you didn't? How did you decide not to run away? What was different?" I was sure that there must be a lot more to this family's story.

There are two tools that I find especially helpful for a quick assessment and definition of the problem: a live family sculpture, if all members are present; or a "behavioral sequence." I decided that at the next meeting we would complete a written behavioral sequence for each time Beth had run away over the past year. At Intensive Family Services, we successfully used behavioral sequencing as one of our assessment tools. If all of the behavioral sequences here were similar, I could merge them into a compilation to review with the family. It was my hope that the insights from this effort might provide us with a strategy to resolve whatever was supporting the runaway behavior so that we could strengthen the family.

A "behavioral sequence" is a circular rendition of behaviors that reveals how one action leads to the next. It illustrates cause and effect, resulting in a specific outcome or even in a recurring pattern over time. It can clarify the *who*, *what*, *why*, and *how*; and can be used in many situations, including law enforcement investigations, family dynamics, and to look at behaviors that reinforce both good and undesirable outcomes. Questions are asked such as:

- "What was the first indication that something was going to happen?"
- "Then what happened?"
- "What happened next?"

The family is providing the information, so they own the sequence of behaviors or events. Each "event" is written down using the family's words with an arrow to the next event until the sequence gives a complete picture, from beginning to end. Cause and effect are thus illustrated clearly on paper in black and white: "This happened→then this→then this." When there is circularity—in other words, when the last behavior or event points back to the beginning—it can be indicative of a pattern. It does not matter where you start on the diagram, as long as you continue to question with, "There must have been something before that?" or "How did it go from here to there?" until you get the beginning, the middle, and the end.

I explained the behavioral sequence process at the meeting that followed, showing them that I was holding a pencil and large sheet of paper. Before we began the process, I emphasized that everyone who was part of these events needed to describe what had transpired. Beth, stepdad, and mom agreed to participate and answer the questions. I referenced the first time Beth had run away and asked: "What was the first indication that something was going to happen, or maybe a problem was brewing?" We went through each of the "What happened? ... Then what happened"? questions and completed the first sequence. Then, I got another sheet of paper and asked about the next time she had run away, and then the time after that. After noting the similarities of each event, the meeting time expired and I set the next appointment, promising that I would have some conclusions and ideas, and that all three of them had to be present. The family agreed to another meeting, each expressing curiosity about what the sequence would indicate.

In between appointments, I compared each of the sequences and looked for both commonalities of events and similar patterns. The sequential maps clearly illustrated causation and a pattern. I developed one sequence to represent all the events. At the next appointment, I would need to process the family's understanding of the compilation and their reaction to it before we could proceed in therapy. The compilation of the sequences looked like this (this would be best illustrated as a circular mapping):

Beth returns home (police, court, or just by herself)→Mom and Beth talk→They agree on consequences/Beth goes to her room "grounded"→Stepdad returns home from work→Stepdad and mom talk→Stepdad and mom disagree on consequences for Beth→Mom and Stepdad argue/gets louder and louder/threats of leaving and divorce→Beth comes out of her room/joins argument→Beth stands between mom and stepdad/Beth and stepdad argue/volume escalates→Other children run to their rooms/some are crying→Beth runs to her room/mom and stepdad continue arguing→Arguing continues on and off for one or more days→Beth sneaks out window or door and runs away/arguing stops/concern for Beth's safety →(pattern continues from beginning).

Arnold, Karen, and Beth arrived early for their appointment, clearly interested in my conclusions and ideas. I asked them, "What's better?" and they told me that things had been calmer, and Beth had not run away that week. We processed their report of improved communication, and I asked about the younger children. Their report was that on Saturday, the family had gone to a fair; and on Sunday afternoon, the children—including Beth—had gone to a matinee. I learned that Beth liked being put in charge as the older sister and "guardian" of her siblings.

We reviewed the sequence of behavior, and Arnold and Karen instantly had the insight that they needed to be "on the same page." They expressed a willingness to work on parenting issues and communication. At that time, the parents were not ready to "own" the possibility that perhaps Beth running away might have served a function, such as protecting the family, especially the younger children. I held several appointments with the couple, and we focused on consistent communication and parenting. I could see that Arnold and Karen truly understood they had couples issues, and during those meetings they focused on cooperation and communication in the marriage, not on the runaway child.

Approximately three months later, the couple reported confidence that their marriage was strengthened, and they were on board as consistent, unified parents. I suggested that we invite Beth to the next appointment. Beth was clearly calmer and reported that things were "1000 percent" better at home. She had not run away while her parents had been attending therapy. Mom told Beth that she was sorry for everything that had happened, and that she and Arnold understood Beth's "cry for help." Arnold remained silent but did not outwardly challenge Karen's statement. At the end of the session, he told Beth, "I can see you have been making an effort, even making good changes, and we appreciate it. You are great with the kids, and they love you. We can all make this work." And they did.

I scheduled a follow-up meeting with them for two months in the future. To my surprise, they brought all the children. I could see that the younger children loved and admired Beth. Both parents had compliments for Beth and reported that they were pleased with how things had worked out. We decided that there was no need for another appointment unless they wanted a "tune up" at some future date. I did not see them again in my office; but I did see them around town several times over the next few years and their self-report was that they were doing well. I saw Beth's name in the newspaper when she graduated from high school and went away to college.

Couples Counseling with Only One Partner Present

Practicing neutrality between the partners and acknowledging the marriage as the client is nearly impossible when you are doing therapy with only one of the partners. If we represent ourselves as the relationship counselor, it is crucial that loyalty to the relationship be unconditional and clearly stated in order to avoid bias and splitting or triangulation. The informed consent for couples counseling needs to state that any disclosure by one of the partners will be shared with the other partner. Conversely, when we are the therapist for the individual, we need to be clear that confidentially and privacy are strictly honored, even if addressing marital issues in individual therapy. As I have previously stated, my conviction is to avoid providing individual therapy and couples therapy for the same client.

When I began my training in marriage and family therapy, the theory was that you could not do marital work with only one of the partners in the room. A decade later, in *Divorce Busting*, Michele Wiener-Davis (1992) pioneered the "it takes one to tango" approach using solution-oriented therapy, developing a niche to work on relationship issues with only one of the partners in session. It is still individual therapy, not a couples session. The idea is to help the client work on issues individually, while clarifying and processing whatever needs to be addressed in the marital relationship, seeking to find resolution. She has normalized the idea that "there is usually one person in the relationship that takes the initiative to iron out relationship kinks" (Weiner-Davis, p. 100). If you like this idea, be certain to study and/or train in these methods before you try to address and resolve an individual client's marital issues. And keep in mind that the foundation of her work requires the exclusive use of solution therapies.

Once you have started work on the marriage with an individual partner, beginning couples therapy would be complicated. Accepting a couple as your client after being the individual therapist for one of the partners is still risky. Remember, no confidentiality between the partners means whatever was shared by one individual must be available to the newly arrived partner—the therapist cannot be the keeper of secrets. That possibility alone could complicate, or even derail things for the couple. There cannot be, "I don't want my spouse to know about this or that I brought it up." It would be best to refer the couple out and, if indicated, to continue to counsel the individual with whom you already have a therapeutic alliance.

You might want to consider issuing a word of caution to your "individual client" who is addressing relationship issues. The last thing a marriage needs is for a partner to come home and say, "My therapist said, 'You need to listen better and get in touch with your feelings.' " A statement like that could very well be heard by the marital partner as, "My therapist said you are a jerk." Our clients need to use discretion when sharing information from their individual sessions. If a client in individual therapy needs clarification or resolution, one option that is available when doing solo work is to use an empty chair to allow your client to "speak to" their partner—at least until marital therapy is possible for them with another provider.

One other thing: anytime you do individual work with a client who is in a relationship, keep in mind the systemic nature of families and the feature of homeostasis. Any change your client makes will have an effect on the partner and the whole family. I would advocate that the therapist asks the question, "When you're doing that [what the client just said they would be doing], what will your spouse/partner be doing?" We owe it to our clients to address how changes will affect the marriage and impact the client's family system. There are always sensitivities and vulnerabilities, and thus the potential to inadvertently cause damage to the marriage and family when working with one of the partners.

Michelle Is Taking Control and Defining What Change Looks Like

A couple of decades ago, a client named Michelle stopped in at my office and asked for an appointment to attend individual counseling. Five years prior, she had attended one of my weekly "codependency" groups for more than a year. Michelle worked as a planner for a national corporation, and I remembered her as organized, determined, and committed to self-improvement. Michelle explained that she had done well for four years after she left the group, but the last year had been "shaky," and she had lost her way. Her children were now teenagers, and she felt that they did not need her as much as they did when they were young.

During the intake session, Michelle was clear that it was time for her to take a stand and get control of her future. Her mindset was that she needed to organize her thinking and identify each step along the way. She also shared with me that she remembered from group that I had said goals come from the client, and the therapeutic relationship is a partnership for change, so she entered therapy prepared to set goals and follow them. Michelle was upfront about her agenda and made it easy for me to decide on an approach. She was asking to set incremental goals and develop a plan as a first step in therapy, so I decided to use a scaling technique in a somewhat modified way to fit her agenda:

Saul: Hey Michelle, let's say a 10 on the scale means your life is the way you want it to be when you have solved the problem that brought you here; and a 0 is how bad things were at the time you decided to see me for an appointment. Where are you now?

Michelle: I am probably a 3.

Saul: Wow—how did you do it? Move up from a 0 to a 3 in such a short time?

Michelle: I had to take charge of things. My life was a mess. I sat my husband down and said we had to talk. He squirmed a lot, but I had a long, serious talk with him.

Saul: Has it been a while, or do you regularly have a talk with him?

Michelle: That was the first time in forever; I can't remember when the last time was that I spoke my mind with him. It was a relief; but afterwards I felt frustrated that I hadn't done it sooner.

Saul: What else did you do to go from a 0 to a 3?

Michelle: I went to two Al Anon Meetings, and an ACOA [adult children of alcoholics] support group. It's been too long since I last went. I saw a few old friends who I haven't talked to in years. It was really good for me. I felt like a new person.

Saul: That's great! I know that's a big step. Good for you! So, what would it take to go from a 3 to a 4?

Michelle: I have marital stuff to take care of. I need to reset my priorities. I guess I would be putting my self-care first and taking a stand with Brad. I'm tired of the stress and uncertainty.

Saul: How exactly would you do that?

Michelle: Keep going to group and detach from Brad's crap. I will be planning things with my friends more and find a sponsor—someone with a lot of wisdom and life experiences. I know that works for me, to have someone out there as a check. It's what I've needed to do.

Saul: When you are a 5—it's maybe a couple of months from now and you have detached, are continuing with group, have a great sponsor, are taking care of your needs, have put your priorities in order—what will be happening to tell you that you are a 5?

Michelle: When I'm doing those things? Well, I think Brad will know it's for real. I need more from our marriage. He will talk to me about what is going on. I think he'll want to know. I will make sure he knows how serious I am; and I will tell him that I won't let him get in the way of my recovery. The kids will notice, and I'll know that I am being a good role model for them.

Saul: When he is taking you seriously, what else is he doing differently that you will notice? And what are you doing differently that he will notice?

Michelle: He will ask me how I am doing more often, and I will stay on track. He will know that I am not backing down because I need to take care of myself to take care of the kids. We will be able to talk more often because I will insist. We'll have a few serious talks.

Saul:	So, what's next? When you are a 6, what will be different and how would I know you are a 6? How will Brad know you are a 6?
Michelle:	I will invite him to couples counseling with me. Brad will be sitting next to me, and we will work on communication and how a loving couple needs to act toward each other. I will no longer feel obligated, and he'll know it. He will need to continue being sober and no more relapses every few years. We will be able to recommit after a while, and both of us will take responsibility for what our children need. I want to stay married but not like this. I deserve better. The kids deserve better.
Saul:	Hey Michelle, that's impressive. You know, that might be a 10 if it goes that way. It's definitely higher than a 6.
Michelle:	I know, I can see that; but I've got to get this done, and soon. I'm fed up—really tired of the same old crap.
Saul:	So, I'm hearing quite a bit about what will be different for your marriage. I'd like to understand more about what the payoff is for you. When you do all those things, what would be different with you?
Michelle:	I will have more confidence in myself. I will look forward to getting up in the morning; will be a good mother to my kids; will see my family more often. I will have a normal life. I want a—like we used to say in your group—a healthy life with fulfillment. My life, my dreams of what my marriage and family can be!

When a client sees how change will happen, it makes success more likely. I have told clients many times, "If you can visualize what the change will look like, you can do it." Michelle set the table for our work together. She had created the map of what progress would look like. I asked, "What's better?" at the start of each session, and then I "threw success in her face." Her description of how things were changing in her direction provided the benchmarks to assess and chart her progress in therapy.

Michelle had also opened the door for couples counseling in the future, and Brad eventually did commit to couples counseling. However, I found it prudent to refer them to another marital therapist. Michelle had been my client both in a process group and in individual work, and it would have been improper for me to attempt to be a "neutral" therapist for the couple. Michelle completed individual work with me over the next six months, and reported that she and Brad had resolved most of their issues in marital therapy by that time. A decade later, they were still married—I know because not too long ago I saw Michelle and Brad, their granddaughter, and their infant great-grandson! Michelle was an exceptional and heroic client.

Couple Issues Can Be Complicated but Are Usually Resolvable

Client-couples have demonstrated that despite the amount or intensity of their arguing, they can find self-control and the means to change their patterns. Changing dysfunctional patterns offers an opportunity to create a new pattern of communication for healthy sharing and resolution. Ironically, for future-oriented therapists, this can mean that the couple will be looking back to a time when things such as communication, energy, fun, and sex were better than they have been more recently. Many couples have lived some of their answers during an earlier time in their partnership.

The stages that relationships pass through are often unique and not readily predictable, but there seems to be commonalities of ups and downs. I have learned that couples universally have periods when things are calm and loving, with the means to communicate without conflict and animosity. Other stages might be described as routine and boring; or conflictive and unhappy. When couples come to therapy, it is often because they are in crisis and concerned about the future of their marriage or relationship. No two couples are going to present their history and dynamics in the same way.

Partners know more than they might think about how to solve their problems and get back on a good track, so therapists need to do a thorough relationship history and ask for exceptions to the presenting problem. It is important to identify strengths and build hope beginning from the first meeting. More often than not, one or both partners are customers over saving their marriage. When couples present as complainants or one presents as a visitor, problem talk often dominates; but that does not mean that there is no silver lining. Even disagreements can be constructive and lead to positive outcomes. A skilled couples therapist does not hesitate to ask, "When have you had a disagreement and something good has come out of it?"

References

Haley, J. (1987). *Problem–Solving Therapy.* 2nd ed. San Francisco, CA: Jossey-Bass, Inc.
Madanes, C. (1981). *Strategic Family Therapy.* San Francisco, CA: Jossey-Bass Publishers.
Weiner-Davis, M. (1992). *Divorce Busting.* New York: Simon and Schuster, Inc.

13 Grief Work

Eliciting Solutions to Overcome Loss and Strengthen Resilience

There are a variety of losses that clients can experience: a death; loss of a job; a relationship breakup or divorce; "empty nest syndrome," occurring when grown children leave home; loss of health or function; material losses due to a catastrophe or natural disaster such as fire or flood; being a victim of crime; and others. Some losses are the consequences of choices, while others are beyond a client's control. My work with clients has taught me the importance of listening carefully to how they define the loss; the impact the loss is having on their lives; what they have tried that did not work, did work, or perhaps worked a little bit; what they think they can or cannot do; what they have learned or done in the past when experiencing a loss; and if they believe there is a meaning to or lesson behind the loss.

Some clients believe that there are stages and feelings common in the grieving process; while others believe that most everything about their experience is unique. Listening to and observing clients suffering from loss has taught me that however an individual defines the meaning and dynamics of their experience tells me a lot about what is important to them and what they need. There are no preset standards in the process of recovery or healing. Each client will personally wade through their individual and unique restorative process on the way to overcoming challenges and healing from losses.

Books or guides that try to normalize stages or processes can be a "double-edged sword" for clients, meaning that they are not necessarily constructive. When clients have disclosed reading a book that told them about feelings and stages, if they accept that information as their reality and it fits with what they are experiencing, I try to work within that frame. The caution is that artificial standards and expectations can cause more distress and even do harm, so I will routinely tell clients that everybody processes loss differently; their experience is unique to them; there is no hard-and-fast timeframe; and they have everything they need to figure it out. Some religions offer rituals or strategies for grieving that can work

DOI: 10.4324/9781003397380-13

well for clients, usually involving participation with and support from friends and family. Some even include a time ceiling for a grief ritual in order to provide a consistent transition into "normalcy" following loss.

I was surprised that colorful metaphors offered by group therapy participants were well received by fellow clients grieving over relationship loss or divorce, addiction relapse, or situational losses. For example, I have heard clients in my groups offer at opportune times: "Depression is living in the past; worrying is living in the future; if you have one foot in the past and one foot in the future, you are peeing on the present;" and, after one member shared a difficult situation or memory without an outward display of emotion:

> You are like a duck. Ever watch a duck go across a lake? Looks smooth as silk on the surface. But if you look under the surface, you see their little feet paddling like hell! Tell us what is under the surface for you.

Feedback in group affirmed that the metaphors offered made sense, stuck with members, and helped them to visualize "the problem." As a clinician, with the responsibility to monitor exchanges, I could see that when offered by peers, the metaphors were usually constructive in moving clients toward solutions.

Overwhelmed by Grief

Grief from the death of a person can be challenging to address, and there is the risk that grief will devolve into complicated grief—a disorder characterized by intense distress that interferes with functioning (Ghesquiere et al., 2011). My personal history connected to understanding and reconciling grief was stunted because my family believed that children needed to be sheltered from death and the grieving process. Even into my early teens, I was not permitted to attend a funeral or be in the presence of grieving relatives. There were several deaths in my family, including two of my maternal uncles. My mother was devastated. I recall her overwhelmed with grief that lingered for many months when her older brother, Paul, died in his mid-30s. Even at 12 years old, I was prevented from being around my grieving relatives who were "sitting shiva." Not being able to participate in and witness the grief process as a child impacted me in several ways professionally.

Throughout my training to be a therapist, and during licensure internships, I would have been uncomfortable addressing a client's grief issues. After a time, I disclosed my apprehension to one of my clinical supervisors, and he suggested that I attend trainings in loss and grief therapy in order to build my skills. I was somewhat hesitant to accept his counsel. He tried to convince me that I had the listening skills and sensitivity to be helpful with clients grieving over the death of a loved one; so I did not believe he truly understood that my Achilles' heel was about *comfort* with clients who had suffered a loss due to the death of a loved one.

I am a strong believer in continuing education and attended many American Association for Marriage and Family Therapy conferences during my private practice years, eventually completing several trainings that addressed counseling for clients who are experiencing a loss. Workshops—even those offering advanced practice skills—would not necessarily make a clinician comfortable or competent in any given clinical area. Looking back, I would say that it was my clients who helped me to be more comfortable with and better understand the uniqueness of the grieving process following the death of a loved one. In particular, an experience for which I was totally unprepared initiated a process that helped me to shed my reluctance around grief work with clients.

Two years after I received clinical licensure, I was providing couples counseling for an intelligent, creative, and compassionate couple, Murph and Carla. Carla's sister-in-law—her brother's wife—had been killed in a car accident several months earlier, and they mentioned that her brother was not coping well. I gave them the name of a grief counselor who had a good reputation; but to my surprise, they brought the grieving brother into the next session and in front of him asked me if I would help with the overwhelming grief he was suffering.

As they had described to me, Bret was overwhelmed and emotionally paralyzed by feelings of emptiness, sadness, and anger over the death of his wife, Faith. A drunk driver had crossed over the centerline and slammed her car off the side of the highway, killing her instantly. Bret presented as distressed and in crisis, clearly in need of "psychological first aid." I agreed to a session with him right then and we rescheduled Murph and Carla in my next opening that week. Bret shared his feelings and the loss of his life's dreams, sobbing at times and standing up to pace around the office with flailing arms. I listened, at times tearing up while supporting him as best I could. The emotion was gripping, and I felt empathetic pain and sorrow throughout my body. I encouraged him to continue to talk about Faith: how they met; their dreams and plans, marriage, activities, likes and dislikes.

During that intake session, and for the next two sessions, Bret continued to talk about his pain and anger over the loss of his wife. Clearly, he was overcome emotionally and knew that he needed to talk about Faith. Bret expected me to listen and support his process, and I did everything I could to validate and comfort him. It was helpful that Bret and I had a strong clinical connection; but I was concerned that his grief could morph into a pathological condition, perhaps clinical depression. I knew that I had to become more than a support and listener—I had to figure out a way to be a catalyst for healing. I had to trust that the more I listened, probed, and tried to understand, the better the chance that Bret would be able to tell me about times he felt a little better and what more he would need.

I asked him, "How do you honor Faith?" Bret reflected for several seconds and then said, "I've never thought of it that way. But I built an altar to her. I have pictures." He opened a small backpack that he carried and showed me pictures of the site of the accident, where several yards off the road he had built a cross, and placed next to it a large dollhouse of Faith's that contained several stuffed animals, including a teddy bear with her name embroidered on it. Behind those items, there was a small stand and shelf that he had built, sheltered under a small awning to protect them from sun and rain. On the shelf were several pictures of them together. Bret told me he visited the site almost every weekend. The place of the accident was about a 90-minute drive each way from his home.

As he talked about his visits to the site, I could see he was getting more tense and teary eyed. His body tightened and he was visibly angry. I asked Bret about his drive there and what was different when he returned home. He said that he wanted to "pound the steering wheel" and "kick out the windows" in the car during the drive home, and it usually took him a day to recover. Bret's explanation of "recover" was that he could slow down and temporarily put aside the tension in his stomach and chest. From our discussion, I was able to gain solid insight into what he had been experiencing and what to process next with him.

I said:

Bret, you've given me some important information and I think I understand better what you have been going through. Losing Faith has been horrible. You shared a beautiful life with her. Clearly, the love that you and she have is still alive in you. Whenever you talk about her and your life together, I can hear the beauty and passion you shared. When you talk about her death, I can see and hear the hurt and anger in your body and words. You have a right to all that hurt and anger. Those feelings belong there when you think about her death, and it sounds like the visits to the place of the collision reminds you of Faith's death instead of the beautiful life you had together. It sounds more about a place that represents Faith's death than a place to honor her life.

Bret responded:

I didn't know; I didn't think about that. I didn't want it to be like that. It's true; yes, I hate that place. Hate it! It was supposed to be a tribute to her. The cemetery is also death, emptiness, and I feel a void inside even thinking about it. I can't go there without becoming even sadder and hurting too much. It's the worst place.

I said, "That makes sense to me. Bret, tell me about times when you think about Faith and feel warm—feel closer to her." He responded:

When I talk to her. I know she's in heaven. For a while writing helped, but that takes too much time and it's frustrating if I don't find the right words or finish. It's better when I talk to her.

I inquired further, "How have you been honoring her life and dreams, and the life the two of you had together? Where and how are you honoring her living memory in a way she would have liked?" Bret focused on the question for a few moments and then said, "She has a garden in our back-yard. It's really nice. It means a lot to her, and I've been keeping it up because I know she would like that." I reflected back his words: "So that sounds like a place where you are honoring her life." Bret agreed, and talked about how he could make the garden more of a place to honor Faith, talk to her, and build a memorial for her. In fact, that's exactly what he did before our next appointment. On his own, without any prompting from me, Bret moved the dollhouse, stuffed animals, shelf, pictures, and awning from the highway memorial to the garden at their home.

Bret came to see me for several more meetings, and I could hear steady progress in his disclosure. He was sharing regularly with family members, including Murph and Carla. Several times he reported that he had a grip on things and although he missed Faith greatly, was able to feel blessed for the time they had together and the memories she left with him. The garden thrived and he had added to the memorial several small statutes and souvenirs from vacation trips that he and Faith had enjoyed together. Murph and Carla told me several times that they were relieved about Bret's progress. Their feedback helped me to confirm that Bret was on track and doing what he needed to heal. During that time, I was noticing more disclosure from Bret about the memories of the good times he had with Faith and how much he missed her, rather than the anger and hurt that had prevailed earlier.

In the end, eliciting from Bret what helped him to celebrate his life with Faith and feel better was one of the keys for him to heal. His idea to build a memorial to Faith was an important part of his solution; but he originally built it at a place that reflected loss instead of a place where he could cele-brate her life. It was important to support the memorial idea and let him figure out that her garden would be the appropriate place to honor her. It came down to indirectly processing a basic exception question: "When do you feel a little better?" I have come to understand that after listening to a grieving client's pain and understanding where they are in the grief process, it is helpful to ask, "How do you honor [your loved one]?" and begin a process to acknowledge what works and/or build tasks with clients to acquire a sense of control, healing, and even closure.

Another meaningful insight I gained indirectly from working with Bret was about the meaning of a funeral in contrast to the traditional practice in Judaism of "sitting shiva." A graveside funeral can function as a way to acknowledge and perhaps accept that death occurred; whereas sitting shiva is a means to remember and celebrate life. For some of us, a gravesite can intensify grief; whereas for others, it can provide meaning and even comfort. No one rule or tendency universally applies to a client. Each client will have to find a personal way to process grief and make sense of things. Being a good friend, relative, or therapist means that we need to have compassion while being nonjudgmental and tolerant of differences in the grief process, offering the space and support to promote personal healing.

As I have gotten older and more open to varying ideas and perspectives, I have come to appreciate that ancient religious teachings often contain a great deal of wisdom and truth about human behavior and emotion. The recorded wisdom of mankind over the last 6,000 years provides a surprising degree of wisdom and insight into the human psyche and the cycle of life. The idea that we need a ritual to accept death, mourn, and say goodbye, and then a process to celebrate the person's life as we build remembrances for appreciation and healing, seems to be fundamental to the healthy human condition.

My experience working with Bret was one factor in reducing my apprehension around providing therapy for clients grieving over the death of a significant other. During the next decade, I worked with a handful of clients who experienced grief over the death of a loved one; although I did not see myself as a "go-to" clinician for grief work. Then my mother unexpectedly passed away from a hospital-borne infection following minor surgery. I experienced all the intensity and feelings of loss and powerlessness that come with grieving the death of the person who had given birth to me, loved me, and cared for me.

Generally, I do not believe that a therapist must have firsthand experience with any particular issue in order to be effective in treating a client. In fact, I know there is a possibility that it can be an impediment. I do acknowledge, however, that my mother's death provided me with a perspective that reduced my discomfort with grief counseling. The workshops that I had completed, coupled with years of clinical experience and then my processing of personal grief, were sufficient for me to feel more confident and willing to assist clients wrought with grief over the death of a loved one. Therapists need to recognize their limits as well as their strengths, informing and either accepting or referring clients appropriately. I was now confident that I had the tools, mindset, and comfort level to understand and be helpful to clients suffering bereavement.

"I Need to Fix Things at Home and My Wife Wants a Note from You"

Not all interventions for loss and grief are routine or clear-cut. Clients can demonstrate behaviors or moods that are the product of unresolved grief long after a loss has occurred. The connection of moods or behaviors to the death of a loved one are often unbeknown to the client, and it can be difficult for a therapist to assess causation. A thorough client culture and history can provide clues, but an understanding of family structure and dynamics is most helpful when developing treatment strategies. A high-functioning, stable, and solution-motivated family member can be a helpful asset to the therapist in making sense of the family puzzle. Richard was that remarkable, gifted client who made a good outcome possible for his family. The particulars of this referral and the family dynamics were uncommon.

One evening, shortly before I switched the office phone over to the answering service, I received a telephone call from a woman asking if I had time to see her husband, Richard, the next day. Generally, I prefer to speak with the client directly about the reason for an appointment and then secure a commitment that they will attend. Cathy, Richard's wife, was insistent about setting the appointment "for him, only for him"; and I agreed after thinking that perhaps there was a personal reason that he was uncomfortable making the call. She promised that Richard would show up on time; but if he did not for any reason, "I will pay you myself for the appointment time." I was intrigued by her persistence, and we set a time for Richard to attend.

Sure enough, Richard arrived at my office on time. He was somewhat uncomfortable and began with an apology:

> I'm sorry if my wife said anything confusing or inappropriate to you. This was her idea, not mine; and it has to do with her mother. She told me to tell you that I need to come home with a note from you. My mother-in-law would probably love it if I didn't come home ever. She's great as a mother to my wife and a grandmother to our kids, but she is awful toward me. She is bitter and cold in her tone, and her stares could kill. She used to treat me well but following the death a year ago of her husband—Cathy's father—she had to move in with us and something changed. She is just mean spirited and short with me, like I did

something wrong; but she won't talk about it. My friends describe her as a classic "battle-axe," but I wouldn't call her that.

I had to smile when he said "battle-axe," and after hesitating for a moment he laughed, which caused me to laugh also. I told Richard that I would try to be helpful but that I needed to hear the whole story, and as my client, what he wanted would be my priority. He appeared somewhat surprised, so I reiterated that he was my client, and I was going to work for him. Richard asked me why I would be required to work for him and not his wife because "this was all her idea—for me to come here and fix things." I explained to Richard that he would be welcome to represent any person's views or ideas, but I would give priority to whatever he stated were his goals. He reflected on my explanation and then said that his goals would not be against his wife's wishes anyway.

Richard told me that his personal reason for coming to therapy was for his children and wife, and that his mother-in-law had pressured his wife to insist that he "get help or get out." Richard said of his home situation:

> Kids should never have to put up with parents and grandparents that fight and speak ill of each other, and so I've remained civil. I let grandma's stuff roll off my shoulders. Grandma's great with Cathy and the children, but I need to figure out how to get her off my back. I make a good living and love the children. I don't get arrested or blow money, and I provide well for my family. My mother-in-law called my boss twice to check on me because I was working overtime and she suspected that I had a girlfriend. And wouldn't you know it, my boss asked me if something is wrong and if I need some help. I can't let that happen in my position. It is all because of her calls that my boss was suspicious.

Richard worked as the chief shop foreman and union representative at a manufacturing plant owned by a large national company. He was a highly decorated veteran and stated that he would do anything for his country and his family. Richard and his wife Cathy had three children: Mandy, 13; Ted, 11; and Trish, seven. He professed strong family values and saw himself as a provider and protector. When Cathy's father passed away about a year before, Cathy's mother had reluctantly moved in with them for financial reasons. Richard described his wife's deceased father as an alcoholic "who couldn't hold the same job for long and drank himself to death." Richard explained that his mother-in-law had never been a warm or compassionate person, but did not cause them problems until her husband died and she moved in. He described her as a "tough, stern woman, who used to sometimes be a 'hard ass' in order to cope with her alcoholic husband for 40 years."

Richard was insightful and talked intelligently about how his wife's childhood had affected her:

> Cathy would be the caretaker for her father, and the comforter and "security blanket" for her mother. Cathy's mother grew up with an abusive father and sought protection from her mother, who was depressed and not emotionally available or protective. We're pretty sure Cathy's mother married young, at 17, to get out of the house; but there was definitely love between Cathy's father and mother, in spite of his drinking. Sometimes Cathy's father acted like he worshipped and honored Cathy's mother, but mostly he just ignored her and took her for granted.

Richard's words and insights sounded well informed, accurate, and sincere. "I just recall the stories my wife has shared over the years, and her emotional reactions have stuck with me," he explained. I took a large piece of paper from a printer roll, and we sketched out a genogram with three generations of his family and his wife's family. The family dynamics on both sides made some sense of Richard's situation. His wife's family history featured alcoholic fathers and caregiving wives and daughters—although Cathy's mother truly loved her husband and for the most part, they had an interdependent and functioning arrangement despite his drinking.

From Richard's family history, it was clear that he played several roles as a child. Initially he was the mascot and peacemaker in his family of origin, yearning to be the hero, holding strong traditional values of work and family. Richard's sister, seven years older, had occupied the hero role when she was living in the family home. She achieved high-school salutatorian and attended an Ivy League university, never again returning to her parents' home. Her contact with her parents was sporadic after she graduated from college and married. Richard recalled that shortly after his sister left home, he and his parents became closer, and they rained praises on him. It pleased his father when he joined the Reserve Officers' Training Course in high school. After graduating with distinction, he enlisted in the military, was honored as a war hero, and went to work in the trades. Richard was a special services member but declined to talk about any of his experiences while serving.

A natural leader, conscientious and well spoken, with sound work and organizational skills, Richard excelled on the job and was promoted to team leader or foreman in each organization where he had been employed. In his current position, he was charged with the responsibility of directing all the company's foremen and sitting on the management advisory committee. His presentation was modest and low key, but confident and intelligent.

Richard had asked me what I was thinking about the note he needed to bring home to his wife. I asked him what the note needed to say for his wife to be satisfied. To my surprise, he said:

My wife just needs to know if therapy can help me figure out how to make things better at home. She thinks of me as a problem solver and hopes that I can make things right for all of us.

I asked him what he wanted out of our time together, and he said (a la Rodney King), "I just want everybody to get along." Then I asked, "What about for you—what do you want for you?" He answered:

I hope that I can find a way to get rid of these problems between my mother-in-law and me. If I knew what to do for things to get better, I would do it. That's why my wife sent me to you and that's why I decided to come. I'm not naïve; I know it will take a small miracle for my mother-in-law to do right by me, but I'm willing to try anything. It's a mystery why and how she has changed her attitude toward me.

I committed that at the end of our first regular session, I would write a note to Cathy.

Richard emphasized that he supported everyone in his family and hoped that his mother-in-law would find happiness. His words were, "Whatever I can do to figure out and be part of the solution is on the table." I asked why Cathy had not come with him. Richard responded:

My wife thinks that her mother would see it as a betrayal and as personal criticism against her and about her marriage and parenting. Plus, I have always been the one to solve the problems and my wife believes I am the best person to tackle this.

Toward the end of the first session following the intake, we talked a little more about Cathy's request for a note. I explained that under current legal protections, I could only give a "note" to Richard if he requested it, and then it would be his decision whether to pass it on. He understood and consented, so I elicited Richard's assistance in writing the note. We collaborated and the note read:

Richard met with me today and we discussed the need for calm, honest dialog and understanding, for the sake of the marriage and the children. He is committed to finding answers that will improve things at home. We are working toward a plan that will involve solutions to strengthen family bonds, security, and happiness for everyone. We would hope that you could attend in the future if your consultation is needed, but we understand your situation and we will ask only if we find it absolutely necessary.

Interestingly enough, I began to think of the note after each meeting as an opportunity to keep Cathy engaged, set goals, and monitor progress. What had seemed an intrusive request from her had become a tool to assist with a positive outcome. Richard was a sincere, emotionally available man, and a dedicated husband and father. The more time he spent in session with me, the more I learned about his exceptional strengths and good character. I told him that he had given me some ideas that might help move things along in a productive direction, and we scheduled appointments during the next several weeks.

Richard had described his father as an "Irish family man and drinker, as my grandfather and great grandfather had been." When I asked him to detail what that meant, he said his father was a man of traditions who believed hard work and family were most important, and drinking was how you coped when you needed to get away from the pressures of taking care of the family and job. Richard's agenda was keeping his job; keeping his wife and mother-in-law happy; and giving his children the "best life ever." He saw his responsibility as making things good with his mother-in-law for the sake of his wife and children, while acknowledging that it was the right thing to do for his mother-in-law.

I normalized some of his home life by stating that families sometimes go through tough transitions and perhaps his mother-in-law was displacing feelings of loss onto him. Richard's response was interesting:

> My daddy used to say, "Don't take your eyes off the prize." This is about happiness and security for my wife and kids. It's up to me to figure this out. My only focus is how to fix this. That's the prize. In the military, I learned to be steady and work toward mission success. I can't get caught up in the pettiness and blaming. I'll listen to anything and think about what you offer if it is about fixing this. If there is something that you're seeing, if it will help—yes, tell me. I want to understand everything about the mission so that I can plan for any contingencies.

It was apparent to me that the best way to proceed was to let Richard take charge. Beyond yielding to him as the expert—which I would have done anyway—I needed to let him assess the reasons behind his mother-in-law's behaviors and attitude, ask the questions, and figure out possible solutions on his own without much prompting. I could hear that Richard was compassionate toward his mother-in-law and wanted her to do well in spite of her aggression toward him, so I trusted that he would be constructive and focused on a good outcome for everyone.

I asked him for some insight into what had changed from his mother-in-law's perspective over the previous year. Richard was astute about her losses. He discussed the death of her husband and her loss of independence when she moved in with them. The house that his in-laws had rented was gone. His mother-in-law had to let go of some of her "comforts" since there was not enough room for everything in Richard and Cathy's house. She had also lost some visual acuity the previous year as well as night vision, so she could no longer drive a car. I also learned that Richard's father-in-law had died a few days before Mother's Day, which was also a week before her birthday, and neither day was acknowledged last year. Richard explained that the one thing—probably the most significant thing—he could admire about his father-in-law was how he would make Mother's Day and birthdays into really special events, with cards, gifts, nice dinners, words of appreciation, and champagne toasts.

I asked Richard about the funeral and how his wife and mother-in-law processed grief. He never saw his mother-in-law cry:

> She did not talk much about it, but I could see the stress and hurt on her face. At first, I thought she was depressed, then angry, then sort of in a trance; and then she just went on as if nothing happened. I tried to get her to talk to me, but she yelled that it was her business how she handled it.

Richard was quiet and pensive for a minute and then said, "I always suspected that she was venting, and I was the target, but I never figured out why, so I wasn't sure if that was so. Now I'm starting to get it."

I asked Richard, "Over the past year, when were things a little better— maybe times when her attitude toward you was better ...?" He cut me off just as I was finishing the question:

> I was just thinking that on Cathy's and the kids' birthdays—actually, even at times on my birthday—she could be really great. We had big celebrations for the kids and Cathy, and she was involved. On my birthday, I recall that she went along with it and had a good attitude that day. So now, with Mother's Day and her birthday coming up, we need to figure something out. This could be the opportunity I've been looking for.

I complimented him on his insight and idea, and then said, "You have a couple of weeks to figure out what to do and then put things into place. Let's get together next week. I'm excited to hear your plan."

Richard was a pro at completing homework! He came in five days later with a detailed plan to celebrate Mother's Day for his wife and mother-in-law, and to celebrate his mother-in-law's birthday in the tradition of her deceased husband. It looked to me that he had covered everything and more than I could have imagined. He also included a tribute to his father-in-law, and a prayer that this family tradition would continue with his children and for generations beyond.

His plan worked well. Mother's Day included flowers for both his wife and mother-in-law; a big breakfast prepared by Richard and the children; and dinner out at a favorite restaurant. Richard and the children also bought a number of gifts that he knew they could use and enjoy. Richard observed:

> It was a perfect day, I think—at least I thought it was and everyone seemed to appreciate it and have a good time. The kids were great, and I was pleased with how things worked out. Cathy was thrilled and my mother-in-law laughed and smiled more than I've seen in years.

For his mother-in-law's birthday, Richard asked Cathy to join in the planning and they decided to throw a surprise party at home, inviting friends of theirs, a couple of relatives, and several of his mother-in-law's friends whom she had only seen sporadically since the death of her husband. They barbequed and served pastries from a bakery that his mother-in-law loved, adding her favorite ice cream flavors to the dessert. Cathy had suggested that they avoid a birthday cake, knowing that her mother had complained about the cakes that were served in the past on her birthday. I would have thought that a "pastries and ice cream" plan might backfire, but it turned out perfectly, according to Richard.

In the next session, Richard shared with me an insight that he had gained from watching and listening to his mother-in-law during the previous two weeks. He surmised that from her perspective, her husband had given her a good life. They had more than an adequate income for her to be comfortable and she always felt safe, in contrast to her childhood experiences at home with her father. She had more "nice things and comfort" than she ever imagined would be possible; although from Richard's perspective, it looked as if she lived very modestly. In spite of her husband's drinking and emotional distancing at times, Richard's mother-in-law felt secure and comfortable. "I can understand that she really loved him," Richard said. I complimented Richard on his understanding and compassion, and told him that there is a term—"functional alcoholic" —that might describe his father-in-law.

Richard reported that his mother-in-law's attitude toward him had softened, but he was concerned because she seemed "sad and bitter to the core." He theorized that she had never finished, or maybe never started, grieving for her husband. I asked him, "So what will need to happen next for her to grieve his loss?" Richard's response was, "I will find out. I am going to have a heart-to-heart with her, tell her that I get how hard all this must be for her, and let her know that I'm there for her." I followed up with, "When you talk to her, what will be different; and what will your wife say?" Richard answered:

> That's what I need to do—I'll do the talking, but I need to have Cathy there. And what will be different is she'll know I really care, and we will not let anything bad happen to her. I'm going to talk to her as I would my best friend. We are going to help her through this.

It came to me just as the session ended that Richard had given himself a task without any prompting from me. I found myself marveling at his wisdom. On the other hand, I also realized that he was taking a risk with this plan, considering his mother-in-law's recent history with him and how unpredictable unresolved grief can be. My belief in my clients as the expert is strong, and I trust their solutions; but at times my concern for them can interfere with my sleep. This was one of those weeks when I tossed and turned several nights.

Richard's next appointment was the following Monday and I obsessed about it throughout that day. As soon as he entered the room, I knew everything must have gone well. Richard, Cathy, and Cathy's mother had the "heart-to-heart" that Richard had imagined. Richard learned that his mother-in-law had been having difficulty accepting her husband's death; that she was concerned about being a burden to Richard by living there; that she feared Cathy and her grandchildren would resent her for being a failure and disappointing them; and that she was mourning more than her husband's death alone. She told Richard that she had nothing meaningful—no personal keepsake or memorial to his life—to possess and by which to remember him. "It's like he has been erased from this world forever. I have nothing of his that means anything. I can't tolerate that."

After hearing the details of their three-hour discussion, I was relieved—and thrilled with how Richard and Cathy had handled things. He shared that hugs and tears had been plentiful throughout their family meeting, and the door for future "heart-to-hearts" was left open. After the full "play-by-play" was presented to me, I asked Richard, "What about the plan to help her heal, to memorialize her husband?" Richard explained:

> We've decided that mom and I would put together a scrapbook of dad's life, with pictures and key dates and things he accomplished—especially how he showed love to her and Cathy. We started to collect things and

sort through pictures and write down dates and places. Even the kids are involved. It'll be great.

This was the first time Richard referred to his mother-in-law as "mom" and his father-in-law as "dad."

I noted that with all that had transpired, it was an opportunity to tell Richard that perhaps it was time for me to discharge him from therapy. We reviewed his original goals, and what he had accomplished. We processed "fast-forward" questions to predict good outcomes that would continue into the future. He was pleased with the way things had gone and I laughingly said, "You have a 'mom' instead of a 'battle-axe' because of your love and commitment to your family. I'll bet I'm the first clinician to ever say those words." We both laughed.

Several weeks later, Cathy wrote me a "note" and mailed it to my office:

I wanted to write this to thank you. I have my mom back and I'm so grateful. We finished the scrapbook. More than 100 pages and it is beautiful. I feel that I know my dad for the first time and I'm proud to be my parents' daughter. They did not have easy lives, but they made a better life for me. It's because of them that my children will have all the advantages and love a child could ever want. I love Richard and always knew what a magnificent man he is, but I think it is a miracle that he was able to figure this out, even with help. We are a family, and we are close. I wish you much happiness and for the same dreams to come true that you have given us.

Hugs,
Cathy

I believe that once a solution process in therapy gains momentum, it continues even after therapy ends. Richard is a vivid and touching example that clients are the experts on their lives and have everything they need to overcome obstacles. His agenda was to make things right in his family for the sake of his children, wife, and mother-in-law. He did not let his personal grievances or anguish get in the way of his goals. It turned out that this family's problems primarily stemmed from his mother-in-law's unresolved grief and issues related to loss; and part of the solution involved finding a way for the family to honor Richard's deceased father-in-law for his strengths and traditions.

Richard reminded me that we should not assume to understand the issues of and solutions for a particular family in advance of our consultations and inquiries with them. He was a remarkable man, bringing a constructive, forgiving attitude with selfless goals rather than merely venting about his mother-in-law. Cathy trusted Richard with their family's wellbeing and taught me that "bring home a note" does not always mean how it sounds!

Reference

Ghesquiere, A., Martí Haidar, Y. M., and Shear, M. K. (2011). Risks for complicated grief in family caregivers. *Journal of Social Work in End-of-Life & Palliative Care*, 7 (2-3), 216–240.

Epilogue: Thanks to My Clients and Colleagues for a Rewarding Career!

I am fortunate to have been part of the mental health profession, teaching college classes in psychology; writing and facilitating behavioral health and addiction treatment workshops for continuing education; consulting for family treatment programs; working as a therapist in private practice, Juvenile Justice, Child Welfare, adult corrections, and inpatient and outpatient mental health facilities; and serving as a clinical manager at Intensive Family Services' research sites.

I am indeed thankful for a rewarding career and a quality of life greatly enhanced by my choice of professions. It has warmed my heart and nourished my sense of purpose and meaning to observe the courage and resilience of my clients, and the impact of their efforts on generations of children, grandchildren, and great-grandchildren. Teaming with individuals and families seeking self-improvement fits with my heartfelt passion for, and involvement in, several humane, moral movements of my time, such as civil rights; the eradication of hate and racism; the elimination of hunger and poverty; and the humane treatment and care of animals. As a dog lover, during my legacy years, animal charities have become my passion and cause *du jour*!

What makes us the therapists who we are? How do we come to believe what we believe about clients and the therapeutic process? How do we conceptualize change and the therapist's role in accomplishing client change? There are many variables, which include our backgrounds, personal histories, and life experiences; classwork, books and professional training; mentors and internships; exposure to ideas and professional concepts, models, and research; unique family cultures, dynamics, and beliefs; firsthand observations and practice outcomes; lessons from trial and error with clients; willingness to be flexible and open to new clinical ideas and approaches; integrity, maturity, and internal strength to let go of the belief that we are the indisputable experts; trust and open-mindedness to really listen to our clients; and more.

DOI: 10.4324/9781003397380-14

The truth is that clinicians are influenced by many situations and circumstances; and our lifetime of experiences or even a recent occurrence can have a profound impact on our work with clients. I have heard concerns that there is some correlation between new client diagnosis and the subject of recent workshops attended by a psychologist. The conclusion offered by the "academic person of influence" who introduced this issue was that, following attendance at a workshop, a psychologist is likely to assign clients a diagnosis consistent with the topic of recently completed continuing education trainings. Whether that is fact or impression, we know that exposure can have a strong influence on our perceptions, expectations, and beliefs.

I have observed as a student, intern, clinician, supervisor, and clinical manager that despite contradictory evidence from direct clinical work, it is not uncommon for therapists to cling to previously held beliefs or perceptions from their personal life experiences or their education and training. Although in an ideal world therapists would be objective and unbiased, we can be subject to confirmation bias, cognitive dissonance, and other influences that cloud our objectivity and sound decision-making. Professors, workshop facilitators, training in a particular clinical model, or research articles can sway our beliefs, perceptions, impressions, and choice of interventions. The most skilled, insightful, and effective clinicians know better. What "works" for that unique client in front of you needs to be more important than what is documented and promoted in a book, research article, or classroom; or by an esteemed colleague. We need to be agents of our clients' desired change—first and foremost, by letting our clients be the experts on what change looks like.

Is "Evidence Based" the Same as What Really Works for Your Client?

For several decades, researchers have been attempting to determine which clinical models and interventions can be designated as "evidence based." Certainly, there is great value in research that looks at certain aspects of human behavior; but mental health research that looks at clinical models, client change process, and outcomes based on a *Diagnostic and Statistical Manual of Mental Disorders* (DSM) diagnosis will have its limitations. Psychotherapy is not a hard science, although some attempt to treat it as such. There are many factors that concern me when I look at behavioral research, including unmeasured variations in the skill of therapists; client selection and exclusion criteria; client satisfaction variables; cultural differences; geography; unintended outcomes not noticed or measured; and other variables. Large swaths of the population can be overrepresented or underrepresented in, or excluded from, studies. And not all the research is even published.

Most of the established clinical models can accurately claim that research shows them to be evidence based; and I have no doubt that, if applied skillfully, widely accepted clinical models can be effective. In fact, I have seen them work; but I am concerned about recent conclusions from some academics that a specific therapy model would be best for a certain diagnosis. Any representation that a particular therapy model is the best or the only appropriate match for a particular diagnosis may disregard important variables that can affect research and lend itself to client blaming when real-world interventions are unsuccessful. If an approach does not fit for a client, the therapist needs to prioritize the needs of the client and alter the approach. I find repulsive the idea that a client is resistant and to blame if they do not succeed in somebody's "brand" of therapy. Dozens of other therapists' clients have been referred to me with the label "resistant," "difficult," or "impossible"; and many—even most—have thrived in therapy!

I would conclude from decades of observation that loyalty to education and training—to one or another particular school of thought and orientation—appears to influence what research takes place and how it is constructed. There also appears to be an allegiance to certain models that is evident in publications, professional organization endorsements, workshops, and research. There can be incentives behind the endorsement of a clinical model. This is not to demean research or researchers, but simply to alert others to be cautious in drawing hard conclusions on how to proceed with any client. Over the past 50 years, I have observed tensions between private practice clinicians, psychiatry, and academia over "what works" in therapy and clinical practice philosophies. We need to prioritize what works for our unique, individual client instead.

An understanding of client dynamics and therapeutic process would suggest one should be skeptical of blindly adhering to certain popular articles, books, and trends. Even the *DSM* undergoes changes—many significant—every few years. In the first chapter, we discussed a time when homosexuality was considered a pathology. Some of what was once regarded as legitimate "best practice" has been discredited, and in many instances now is categorized as harmful. For example, it was not that long ago when many mental health professionals believed "lost memories" were the root of dysfunction, anxiety disorders, and depression for many clients. Well-regarded clinicians and educators wrongfully supported the concept of behind-the-scenes "lost memories" and the need to intervene with adults to address their "forgotten" victimization as children.

Over the years, children with behavioral challenges in the child welfare, juvenile justice, mental health, and local school systems were given the "trendy" childhood psychiatric diagnosis of the time—the 1980s and 1990s featured attention deficit hyperactivity disorder/attention deficit disorder; and just prior to 2000, the next generation of our child population were labeled as "bipolar"; and children were routinely medicated even with "off-label" and adult psychotropic medications to control their behaviors. We saw the negative repercussions of those interventions as the children entered puberty and then adulthood. These were children who had been traumatized: abused, neglected, shuffled from place to place, suffering loss after loss, the keepers of horrific secrets, with few options but to act out their feelings in a desperate cry for help. No hugs. Little compassion. Few solutions. We need to do better!

Therapists, take a breath! Disregard the static! Focus on what works for the client in front of you. What is it they want from therapy? What is the payoff for them? How will they know that they don't need to come any-more? What is it they want to be different? What else? When has some of that happened before—even a little bit? How did they do it? What needs to happen for them to do more of it? What will the first sign be that it is beginning to happen? Then what?

Therapy needs to be more about being in a collaborative therapeutic relationship with your client and pushing aside all the trends, obstacles, and craziness! Look at your client's system. What else can you do to tilt things in their favor? Make it happen! Make a difference!

The Legacy I Hope to Leave

I still get emotional and teary-eyed when I recall good things that have happened for my clients, just as I envisioned I would when I began my studies. Even writing and then reading the familiar client stories in this book at times brought tears to my eyes. I am thrilled for my clients, whether their desired change has occurred with me as a catalyst or even sometimes despite mistakes I have made that were corrected by my clients. There are many reasons that I like the unique way of thinking at the core of solution work. The bottom line is that a solution-oriented, strength-based, client-centered philosophy means that I maintain values that enhance client-therapist cooperation, empower clients, and make interaction open and more effective. Success becomes a self-fulfilling prophecy that begins with the collaborative therapeutic alliance. Knowing that what I expect will influence the results, my assumptions focus on my client's strengths and solutions (O'Hanlon and Weiner-Davis 1989, p. 34). Clients are univer-sally regarded as important and "worth it" because they are. For these and other reasons, clients more often embrace the therapeutic process.

The payoff has been the successful discharge of most every client; and now I have been meeting the grandchildren of many clients who had progressed from overwhelmed and struggling into celebrators of life. For many years, hardly a month went by without a contact from a past client or client family. In a grocery store, department store, city park, downtown mall, or post office, individuals or families whom I did not immediately recognize approached me:

> I remember you. I was eight or nine when my parents took me to family counseling. You saved our family. This is my daughter and my grandchildren. I also have a son who is a high-school teacher. My parents always talked about how thankful they were to have you as their counselor.

My response, often through tears of joy, would be something like: "Your parents were the heroes. Really, you need to thank them. It's not about what I did. They were courageous and loved you too much to let anything get in the way of your future."

I also have occasionally received emails or texts from previous clients. These inadvertent meetings and unexpected messages bring me joy and affirm a message I want to pass on. For years, I have told interns and therapists in classes and workshops that their work is important and will have an impact on society and families for many generations to come. Sometimes I share stories about my chance meetings with former clients and their children and grandchildren to help attendees imagine the magnitude of their clinical work. I emphasize in every case that credit goes to the clients for their courage, and for teaching me how to be helpful. Decisions and the effort to make changes are never easy. I also tell them that the few who did not meet their goals might have succeeded if I had understood better how to approach them; but I was not the right person for them, or it was not the right time.

Throughout this book, you have read about various interventions that empowered clients to pull a solution rabbit out of the metaphorical hat! My advocacy for client-need-driven solution work, as a best practice intervention, is because it is about what really works for our clients. Clients define the problem in their own words and identify how incremental change will look. Question sequences encourage client feedback and direction. Therapy is meant to be enjoyable for both the therapist and the client. The therapeutic alliance is strong, based on listening, acceptance, mutual respect, identifying client strengths, and true collaboration. Exceptions to the problem are central to finding solutions. Desired change happens early in treatment and right before the therapist's eyes! And because the client owns the goals and the change process, change is more often real, meaningful, and lasting—not merely compliance or temporary change. Simply put, it really works for a client because it is not a rigid model, but about doing whatever works for that particular client!

Most clinicians I have encountered would say that their early career began with an allegiance to a particular clinical model and philosophy.

Many then attended training over the years that altered some of their thinking, and eventually evolved toward another model or a more flexible approach. Witnessing firsthand the work of several hundred clinicians, what the handful of great therapists I have observed had in common was a toolbox full of techniques, neurolinguistic language ideas, process questions, tasks, and "therapeutic tricks." Each had allowed their early thinking to be challenged, learned to stop blaming clients, and instead modified their interventions to match what actually worked. They discovered that the keys to success include respecting clients as the experts on their own lives and being fans of whatever interventions work for each unique client. Competency is not always about the process; more than anything else, it is about the outcome.

During these legacy years, my hope is that I can pass on to younger therapists and students some of the ideas that I have found helpful. Into my 70s, I have continued to teach continuing education workshops for mental health professionals. Recent topics include ethics; culture and diversity; enhancing outcomes for clients with challenging or unique issues; solution-focused brief therapy; and brief solution-oriented family therapy. The workshops help to connect me to younger therapists, interns, and students, as well as providing me with an understanding of the direction mental health services are taking. I often include client stories in my workshops as a teaching tool to make intervention ideas real and engaging. My parting message to those who attend the workshops, and now to those of you who are reading this, is: your families are depending on you. Generations are depending on you. *Make a difference!*

See Appendix J for a discussion of "constructivism."

Reference

O'Hanlon, W. and Weiner-Davis, M. (1989). *In Search of Solutions*. New York: Norton.

Appendices

Appendix A: New Age Founders

Sal Minuchin, M.D. was a powerful force in structural family therapy, sometimes referred to as the father of family therapy. He was revered for creative interventions, acknowledging client strengths, and offering powerful questions to promote self-reflection and behavioral change. Minuchin's classic language was complimentary, even under duress. I recall hearing him say things like, "Yes, but we know better" to an audience of peers; and "Yes, but you are better than that" to a client. He was a force at the Child Guidance Clinic in Philadelphia, and later opened a training and consultation institute in New York City that he named Family Studies.

Maurizio Andolfi, M.D. was a creative structural family therapist whose work was interactive and entertaining, producing immediate changes in the parent-child hierarchy with one session. He believed strongly in listening to the children in the family. Andolfi moved family members into physical positions that represented the family structure and hierarchy, and then used their insight and discomfort as catalyst for change. He was one of several prominent Italian family therapists. (In Chapter 8, I illustrate the use of his methodology with a family.) I recall hearing from him that Italy held family therapy in such high esteem that it required therapists who worked with families to be licensed medical doctors in addition to holding advanced degrees and certificates in family psychotherapy.

Luigi Boscolo, M.D. and **Gianfranco Cecchin, M.D.** were Italian clinicians who broke with the psychoanalytical mainstream. This team eventually became known, after the separation from Mara Selvini, as the Milan Approach. They developed their practices in Milan, under consultation of Gregory Bateson of the Mental Research Institute (MRI). This break with psychoanalysis and the implementation of family therapy, under the influence of Bateson, was groundbreaking. Outdated, harmful ideas regarding schizophrenia were one of the targets of their earlier research.

Steve de Shazer and **Insoo Kim Berg** founded the Brief Family Therapy Center and developed solution-focused brief therapy, a constructivist approach that emphasized a client's strengths and problem-solving skills. Clients were considered experts in their domain, and therapists elicited solutions instead of telling clients what to do. Their approach includes neurolinguistics that presuppose change and empower clients. Question sequences that take clients beyond their problems, envisioning solutions and the future, are a core skill required of therapists. Their bottom line—which is often omitted or not understood by educators and work-shop facilitators—is that therapists need to do whatever works for the client. Many renowned therapists, researchers, and authors—notably Bill O'Hanlon (possibilities/solution-oriented therapy)—are disciples of their constructivist thinking.

Jay Haley and **Cloé Madanes** were developers of strategic therapy and strategic family therapy, creating interventions around the client's symptoms with directives that resulted in clients ultimately doing what they wanted or what they needed to do in order to facilitate intended change. Understanding and addressing the function of the behavior was their forte, and was at the core of their interventions. They were strongly influenced by Murray Bowen and Milton Erickson. Their model is some-times referenced as a "problem-focused" strategic methodology.

Virginia Satir wrote *Peoplemaking*, a groundbreaking book for both clinicians and clients that looked at the role our families play in making us the persons we are. She was a master at explaining and understanding feelings, and she coined the term "leveling." One of her major contributions was an understanding of the family and the influences of family functioning over generations. Her ideas to achieve self-awareness, self-understanding, and healing are widely accepted.

Milton Erickson, M.D. believed that clients are competent and have every-thing they need to solve problems and live their solutions. Erickson was known as a creative and bold thinker, especially in his time. He saw his role as helping clients to use their own strengths and resources. Erickson demonstrated that through intervention and client tasking, the problem itself could be "tweaked" to become part of the solution. He was famous for his "hopeless client" success stories. Reading stories about his client interventions, such as the African Violet Lady, gives insight into his "outside-the-box" thinking. Erickson is considered an originator of many strategic solution therapy ideas and concepts.

Richard Fisch, M.D. is known for his work in communications and neurolinguistics, and is credited to opening the door to the emergence of brief therapy through the use of words and questions that facilitate real change in only a few sessions.

Gregory Bateson is known as the pioneer of the double bind theory of schizophrenia, and was one of the first to think about families as systems.

Murray Bowen, M.D. is well known for his work at MRI. He is the pioneer of family systems theory. Although the word "theory" comes from the original writings and research, it is hardly theoretical that families are systems, with rules, roles, relationships, and a hierarchical structure.

Paul Watzlawick, Ph.D. was a co-founder of the MRI Brief Therapy Center (with Weakland and Fisch), and is remembered for his research in communication theory and constructivist concepts. He is recognized as an advocate of the brief approach and family therapy. He was one of the first to address the idea that people often create their own suffering when they try to fix their emotional problems.

John Weakland was one of the early advocates and researchers in family systems therapy and brief therapy. His roots include being a student and researcher of Milton Erickson.

Appendix B: Dynamics of Change

Compliance: Obedience while facing the threat of a consequence with a reasonable belief that one might get caught. There might be a formal court order, threat of divorce, or fear of harm that encourages obedience. Compliance is not a bad thing—but it is probably only temporary, related to a threat or fear, and is not real, lasting change.

First-order change: Change that is external and thus temporary. It often looks like real change but is not lasting. Clinical interventions or guidance that "tells" a client what to do can result in behavioral change without internalization, so the change would not be expected to be permanent. First-order change might be regarded as situational.

(Compliance and first-order change in some cases can manifest as "fake it until you make it." Over time, with the right intervention, either can evolve into permanent, internal change; although recidivism is the most common outcome.)

Second-order change: This is permanent, internal, and authentic; whereas first-order change is only situational. Internal change usually results from free choice and a client's genuine investment in the change. A collaborative therapeutic alliance and processes to elicit client goals and solutions can produce internal change more rapidly than would be accomplished with traditional therapeutic models.

Appendix C: Positions Clients Can Take Toward Therapy in General or Issues in Therapy

Visitors do not think they have a problem. They do not know why they are there or what the value of the meeting might be. They seem indifferent; it's not their idea to receive services. A visitor will not do observational or behavioral change tasks, set authentic goals, or accept that participating in therapy will be worthwhile. The fact that they showed up matters and deserves a compliment from you. It is important that we use early session strategies with visitors to motivate them to come back for another meeting.

Complainants have a problem that cannot be solved. They complain about circumstances or other people. It is somebody else's fault. They are good at describing what is wrong but are challenged to find what makes it better. Complainants are great observers and will do observational tasks, but not behavioral change tasks. Working with complainants by listening, validating their concerns, acknowledging their strengths, identifying exceptions and what change will look like, and learning about their agenda(s) will build a solid therapeutic foundation.

Customers have a problem they are trying to solve and are willing to work to change something. Working from their agenda(s) will keep them engaged as customers. Customers will do both observational and behavioral change tasks. We can usually move clients into a customer position through client-centered, client-need-driven solution work that prioritizes their agenda and builds a therapeutic atmosphere and collaborative relationship.

Appendix D: Medical Model vs. Constructivist Thinking

The traditional "problem-focused" paradigm, sometimes called the "medical model," differs in philosophy and practice from the solution-oriented/constructivist model.

Traditional Problem Focused (Medical) Model

- Problem-focused models look to a "professional expert" to identify problems and design the solution. Only the client, who is seen as responsible for their situation, implements the solution. Disagreement with the "professional expert" is called "resistance."
- Problem-focused/medical models assess the presence of "deficits" and determine a course of treatment that may directly address those deficits.
- In the "problem-focused" model, the "professional expert" knows more about and understands the problem and solution more thoroughly than the client.

Solution-Focused (Constructivist) Model

- In the social constructivist or "solution-focused" model, the relationship between the client and the "professional" is collaborative. The clinician is not seen as the sole diagnostician.
- Clinicians notice the client's strengths and resources as opportunities, rather than only focusing on deficits and barriers. The client participates and collaborates with the "professional" in the assessment, the treatment process, and the implementation of solutions.
- Solution-focused processes and assessments allow the "professional" to work with the client "in the environment," beginning from where the client starts, using the client's own words, understanding the client's goals, and building on the client's experiences and successes.

- The "solution-focused professional" explores the client's/family's strengths and expertise, and empowers the family (more as a catalyst than as an expert).
- The "solution-focused professional" offers cooperation with the client, rather than demanding cooperation from the client, adjusting to and respecting the uniqueness of the client and the client's cultural and ethnic traits.
- The "solution-focused professional" uses their skill or knowledge to create a process and in doing so, collaboratively generates and co-constructs solutions that will help the client move toward the desired outcome that represents the client's agenda.
- Research is clearly demonstrating that the social constructivist model produces significantly better outcomes as well as authentic changes that last (second-order change).

Appendix E: Process Questions Following a Setback

Here are some generic questions to help clients build hope and put the current setback (or if there have been multiple setbacks over time) into perspective:

- "How is this setback different from the last one?"
- "What did you do that is different this time?"
- "How did you decide to come here today?"
- "Who did what differently this time that helped?"
- "What do you suppose your spouse [children/parole officer/boss] would say is different about you this time?"
- "What do you need to do in the future to maintain the change you want?"
- "What difference will it make to you when you do this?"

It is also important to find ways to process the positives from the experience through "recovery questions," such as the following:

- "What have you learned about yourself from this episode?"
- "What has this episode taught you about your [drinking] problem?"
- "What will you do differently as a result?"
- "What do you need to do more of?"
- "How will you make sure that you do that?"
- "How do you suppose that will affect your life?"
- "What do you suppose you spouse [children/probation officer/boss] would say you need to do more of?"
- "What difference would it make in your relationship with your spouse [children/probation officer/boss] if you did more of that?"
- "What do you think your spouse [children/probation officer/boss] would do in response?"

Appendix F: Definitive and Possibility Statements, Coping Questions, and Compliments

Definitive statements represent something a client wants to happen and are co-constructed using the word "when"; changing the tense; using qualifiers of time or intensity; adding terms such as "yet" or "so far"; and restating a problem as a goal. Examples might include the following:

- "<u>When</u> things are better, who will notice first?"
- "<u>When</u> you are able to tell her what you want, what exactly will you say?"
- "You haven't gotten much understanding <u>yet</u>. So, what will you be noticing first?"
- "Your efforts haven't been recognized <u>so far.</u> When they are recognized ..."
- [Client complains that no one will hire them] "Oh, so you want to find a job ...?"

Possibility statements imply "if" a problem were to happen again, the client would know how to handle it. Generally, the word "if" is used in conjunction with a question about how the client will handle the problem now that they are better equipped to deal with it. Examples might include the following:

- "If it were to happen again, what would you do differently this time?"
- "With everything you know now, and all your strength and resolve to make this marriage work, if that were to happen again, how would you handle it?"

Coping questions are used when other methods have not provided exceptions or when a client indicates hopelessness. Coping questions are sometimes regarded as the "last resort" for disparaged clients. When coping questions are used properly and appropriately followed by compliments, they can initiate a process that increases client participation and hope. Examples might include the following:

- "How come things aren't worse?" Followed up with a sequence of questions such as:
- "Wow—despite your [client's words], you decided to move ahead; how did you find the strength to do that?"
- "What is it about you that you survived?"
- "How did you cope with that?"
- "How did you find the will to do that?"

Examples of compliments that can be given after a positive client experience with a coping question could include the following:

- "I'm really impressed by your survival skills";
- "You must have a strong will to succeed"; or
- "You must really love your children."

Appendix G: Solution Question Sequences

Solution Process Questioning

- After problem talk, ask for exceptions:

  - "Tell me about a day that was better/a little bit better."
  - "There must have been a time when you were able to get that to stop—even for a little while?"
  - "You said Tuesday was a good day. What was different on Tuesday?"

- "How did you do that?"
- Give compliments.
- "What will be happening next that will tell you that you are on track"?
- "How has this already started to happen, just a little bit"?
- "What else might you do/need to help you get there"?

(Ask coping questions if you are not able to elicit an exception: "How come things aren't worse?")

Goal-Setting Process

- Ask goal-setting questions (i.e., fast-forward, scaling):

  - "On a scale of 0-10, with 0 being the worst it has ever been and 10 being how you want it to be, where are you now?"

- Anchor with a detailed description of behaviors in the client's control:

  - "When you are a 4, what will be different? Then what will happen next?"

- Process with the client. Include "What will be different?" questions for family members and others.
- "How has this already begun to happen, a little bit"?

- Continue to follow process and set incremental goals to the next number on the scale.
- Identify several goals from this process with the client and have the client prioritize goals.
- Use the client's words. Set small increments, likely to be accomplished within three weeks.
- Elicit/assign tasks.
- Scale willingness and confidence to do tasks until they reach 9 or 10.

Scaling Process

- Identify issues.
- Ask, "On a scale of 0-10, where are you today?"
- Scale 0-10 (use the scaling process: "Exactly what makes you a 3 ...?")
- Anchor with a detailed description of behaviors in the client's control that would clearly distinguish it as an increment represented by 3 on the 0 to 10 scale.
- Ask, "When you are [one increment higher], what else will be happening?"
- Make sure that each increment is a small step, achievable within three weeks and within the client's control.
- Have the client describe a change that indicates they will have moved up one increment.
- Ask, "How has that already started to happen?"
- Follow up with:

  - "Wow, you're almost there—how did you do that?"
  - "What else might help you to get there sooner?"
  - "How will I know when you're there/what will you be saying?"

General Guidelines

- If the client identifies what they do not want, ask, "Instead of ... what do you want to happen?"
- Use specific behavioral descriptions, not labels such as "self-esteem"/ "codependency"/"attention hyperactivity deficit disorder."
- Assume progress is already happening. Ask, "How has that already begun to happen?"
- Follow up with process questions:

  - "Wow, you're almost there—how did you do that?"
  - "What will happen that will tell you that you are on track?"
  - "What might help you to get there sooner?"

- Assign tasks to complete increments. Tasks should focus on the client's solution/what the client has asked for.
- Scale willingness and confidence to complete the tasks, negotiating until 9 or 10.
- If the client does not do a task, ask:

    - "What part of task the did you do?"
    - "What did you do instead?"

Appendix H: Child Welfare Culture Predominates

The Child Welfare workshops for several county and state child welfare and mental health agencies that I presented under contract following the end of my tenure with Intensive Family Services, between 2002 and 2016, were followed by live sessions with their most challenging families. Innovations to language, approaches, case planning, goal setting, and crisis intervention were discussed, roleplayed, and demonstrated in-vitro. My contract included individual time with every Child Welfare supervisor and unit in two urban counties and rural statewide offices. Child Welfare staff selected the families for child and family team meetings. Each unit was coached through live practice sessions and home visits with selected families on their caseloads. Clearly, those families did significantly better, and the processes reduced crisis, risk, and recidivism by the agency's own measures. It happened right before their eyes; yet two years after the training, there was regression in child welfare practice at those sites. Child Welfare has many dedicated, committed, and hardworking staff. But there are also staff who act punitively, posture more as law enforcement than social work, and refuse to implement family-centered practices. Perhaps some Child Welfare managers never felt that they owned the changes asked of them; but whatever the reason, some in key positions did not consistently enforce the changes in practice.

A national trainer and court-appointed monitor who for more than 30 years assisted Child Welfare agencies with consent decree compliance in several states told me:

> It has become clear to me that child welfare training is a waste of money. The Child Welfare League of America, Systems of Care, and other resource programs that provide support and training for child welfare have for many decades offered trainings, skill building, and manuals for Child Welfare staff. I've been doing this compliance work for over 30 years. They do not want to "get it" and will never be compliant with

best practices. The only way to get them to follow their own policies and do what's best for kids and families is to instead use that training money to hire an attorney for each family and make sure those attorneys know child welfare law and policies. That's the only way we'll ever fix child welfare.

I hope that is not true!

It is understandable that Child Welfare staff can feel singled out and underappreciated. The culture can discourage workers because it can allow negative thinking to fester; focus on problems and vulnerabilities instead of strengths and possibilities, burden underappreciated workers with excessive caseloads and few resources; and too often choose cynicism over hope. Many Child Welfare staff and supervisors view new trainings as another burden on them. Lawmakers do not fund enough line staff positions to make caseloads manageable. We know that traditional methods in Child Welfare can have a detrimental effect on children and families, and families under their jurisdiction often become discouraged. To improve outcomes, at least in the short term, it might be feasible for them to maintain a separate family-centered, strength-based unit like we had with Intensive Family Services—if only there was funding.

On the bright side, several community mental health agencies embraced the solution focused family-centered ideas and continued to provide staff with advanced training over the next 15 years. Their clinical staff appreciated best practice ideas that helped create strong therapeutic alliances and resulted in desired outcomes with clients. I was able to contract with them for a series of solution-focused brief therapy/brief solution-oriented family therapy workshops to enhance their skills with high-risk, low-resource families who faced challenges with mental illness and addiction.

Appendix I: Learn, Listen, Believe

We have discussed methods, strategies, and techniques to help clients visualize and express what change looks like for them and achieve the outcome they want. Powerful language ideas with exception questions, fast-forward questions, and coping questions help to move the process along. But the most important intervention method involves listening and learning from clients, and prioritizing what the client really wants.

Learn from the client:

- Family
- Culture
- History
- Elicit instead of telling
- Their definition of the problem
- How change happens for them
- What they really want
- Exceptions to the problem that they are already experiencing
- Prioritize and respect their agenda

Listen:

- No judgment
- No analysis
- Repeat their words
- Use their words to describe the problem
- Use their words to characterize and define the solution
- Show understanding
- Show acceptance
- Show empathy, caring, and concern
- Share joy

- Ask about and listen for exceptions to problems
- Acknowledge successes and achievements, even small ones
- Cheerlead efforts and when successful, follow with compliments
- Empower clients
- Believe in them
- Give them what they want whenever possible
- Give them credit for what they have done
- Acknowledge hard work, good intentions, and effort
- Help them to recognize increments of change and new possibilities
- Emphasize how difficult things were and how courageous they've been!

Believe:

- Clients have everything they need to solve problems
- Clients are experts in their domain
- Strengths can be used to overcome problems

Appendix J: Making Sense of "Constructivism"

Clinical models will have a philosophical basis within a "school of thought." There are several schools of thought with varying perceptions, tools for intervention, and advocacy for their clinical models. Evolving from new ways of thinking about how we learn and reason, schools of thought such as constructivism and constructionism have taken a more prominent position in studies. Solution-focused and solution-oriented therapies have a philosophical basis in constructivism.

Advocates of client-centered, strength-based ideas view the relationship between the client and professional as a joint venture. The clinician offers cooperation with the client, adjusting to and respecting the client's uniqueness, cultural and ethnic traits, and pace. Work begins from where the client starts, using the client's own words, understanding the client's goals, and building on the client's experiences and successes. The clinician notices the client's strengths and resources as opportunities, rather than only focusing on deficits and barriers. The client is regarded as the expert in their domain and collaborates with the "professional" in the assessment, treatment, goal setting, and construction of solutions. Behaviors are assessed and described rather than labeling the client with a diagnosis. The professional uses their skill and knowledge to co-create a client-centered solution process to motivate and empower the client to implement solutions that will move the client toward the desired outcome.

Constructivism is the foundation for solution-focused and solution-oriented therapy concepts and processes. Constructivists believe that knowledge is built upon other knowledge; people construct meaning; learning is contextual; and we learn in ways connected to things we already know. In addition, learning is personal and based on our own experiences, so how people learn and the things they learn from some experiences may be different from others. Ideas in the solution process that would be congruent with constructivism include viewing the client as the expert who is capable and has everything that they need; using their words in the definition of the problem; validating the client's experiences; transitioning from problem talk to exceptions and solutions; respecting the client's position and agenda; emphasizing strengths over deficits; asking fast-forward questions; eliciting goals and solutions from the client; acknowledging change with compliments; and, strategically using client-need driven tasks.

Solution therapies are open to creativity and individual client needs, with an emphasis on whatever works for a particular client. Solution work is not a hard-and-fast model but rather a way of thinking, viewing, conversing, and doing. Therapy begins with respecting the client as the expert and listening. I have learned from my clients that the processes work well so long as we are open to listening to and following the client's expertise in identifying goals and solutions. The idea is to use proven language, questions, and processes as they fit for the unique culture and life experiences of a client. Letting clients teach us and prioritizing whatever works for the client in front of you is best practice. Interventions should be customized for each client. Solution work can be brief not by design, but because if administered properly, problem resolution is possible in fewer sessions than many other therapies. If resolution is not progressing quickly, the solution mantra is to do something different until we find what works for our client. Client feedback is golden!

Index

Printed in the United States
by Baker & Taylor Publisher Services